Short-Answer Questions and MCQs in Anaesthesia and Intensive Care

2nd edition

Adrian Dashfield MB ChB FRCA MD
Consultant in Anaesthesia and Pain Management
Honorary Clinical Research Fellow,
Peninsula Medical School
Derriford Hospital Plymouth, UK

Peter M Murphy MB BS MRCP FRCA
Consultant Cardiothoracic Anaesthetist
Derriford Hospital, Plymouth, UK

A
ARNOLD

A member of the Hodder Headline Group
LONDON

First published in Great Britain in 1995
This edition published in 2004 by
Arnold, a member of the Hodder Headline Group,
338 Euston Road, London NW1 3BH

http://www.arnoldpublishers.com

Distributed in the United States of America by
Oxford University Press Inc.,
198 Madison Avenue, New York, NY10016
Oxford is a registered trademark of Oxford University Press

British Library Cataloguing in Publication Data
A catalogue record for this book is available from the British Library

Library of Congress Cataloging-in-Publication Data
A catalog record for this book is available from the Library of Congress

ISBN 0 340 807083

1 2 3 4 5 6 7 8 9 10

Commissioning Editor: Serena Bureau
Development Editor: Layla Vandenbergh
Production Controller: Deborah Smith
Cover Design:Nichola Smith

Typeset in 10.5/13pt Berling Roman by Servis Filmsetting Ltd, Manchester
Printed and bound in Malta.

What do you think about this book? Or any other Arnold title?
Please send your comments to feedback.arnold@hodder.co.uk

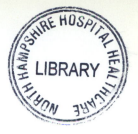

This book is dedicated to our wives Sue and Jo. Without their support and encouragement this project would have been impossible.

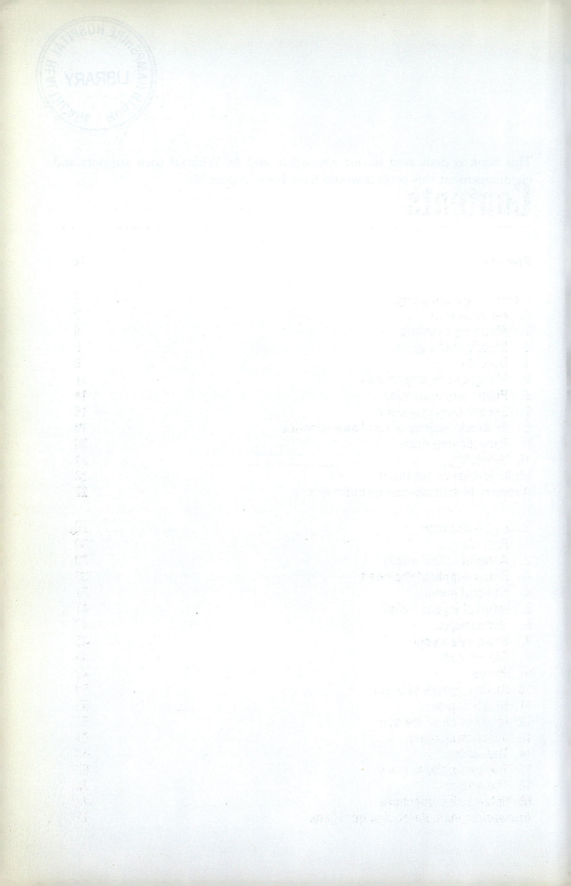

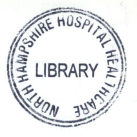
Contents

Preface

This book was originally intended to be a second edition to *Essays and MCQs in Anaesthesia and Intensive Care*. The introduction of the compulsory short-answer question (SAQ) in place of the longer 40-minute essay in the final FRCA examination in 1996 forced a complete rewriting of the text.

This book takes a question-orientated approach. This is not a textbook of anaesthesia. Instead this is an exam-orientated guide. One of our aims is to introduce methods and systems of answering questions succinctly and accurately. The questions have almost all been asked in the final FRCA since 1996. The syllabus is extensive and build-up to the final FRCA must be viewed as a six-month campaign. Hard work must be guided in the right direction, however, as good examination technique is essential to pass this hurdle. Because all twelve SAQs must be attempted with 15 minutes allowed for each SAQ, previous practice at writing SAQs prior to sitting the examination is essential.

The questions here are structured as if for a written or oral answer of the standard required in the final FRCA. There is often more detail than required to reach a pass standard.

Each of the twelve sections has a part containing multiple-choice questions (MCQs) of a similar standard to those set by the Royal College of Anaesthetists. It is vital that candidates practise MCQs as well as SAQs. The 90 multiple-choice questions that follow the SAQ paper carry just as much weight as the SAQ paper. Candidates seem to breathe a sigh of relief and relax over lunch prior to sitting the MCQ paper in the afternoon. Although there are not the same time pressures in the MCQ examination, it is advisable not to take this paper lightly!

Note regarding drug names

We have included in this edition the names currently in use for drugs. However, we do appreciate that new names for certain drugs are currently being phased in, in line with international guidelines. Examples appearing here include:
lignocaine to lidocaine;
methohexitone to methohexital;
thiopentone to thiopental;
trimeprazine to alimemazine.

Adrian Dashfield
Peter Murphy
May 2004

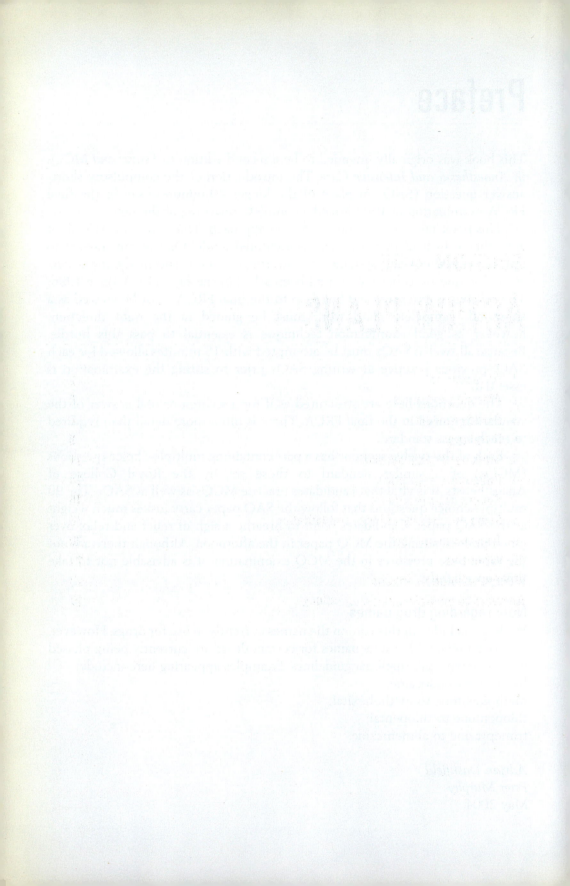

SECTION ONE

ACTION PLANS

1 Air embolism

> Describe the management of a patient you suspect of having developed intraoperative air embolism.

Air embolism is an iatrogenic ingress of air into the vascular system. Air is by far the most common gas which may cause embolism. However, embolism may occur following use of other gases such as carbon dioxide (laparoscopy) and nitrous oxide. Venous air embolism is most common. Arterial air embolism can occur as a result of air crossing into the systemic circulation via heart defects or pulmonary shunts. Other causes of arterial air embolism involve direct cannulation such as in cardiac surgery or angiography.

Air embolism should be suspected in any operation where large veins are exposed above the level of the heart; e.g. thyroid, mastectomy, head and neck surgery. *Confirm* if possible. Can bubbles be seen in the wound? Can froth be squeezed from the veins?

Signs and symptoms

* There is visible evidence of air being sucked into veins.
* Significant embolism leads to tachycardia, hypotension and tachypnoea.
* There is gasping respiration (if breathing spontaneously). A 10% obstruction to the pulmonary circulation can cause a gasp reflex.
* There is an unexplained fall in end-tidal (ET) CO_2 due to an increase in physiological dead-space and intrapulmonary shunting.
* ECG abnormalities described include signs of right ventricular strain, atrioventricular block, tachyarrhythmias, ST segment elevation or depression, and non-specific T-wave changes.
* There is an unexplained fall in blood pressure or dysrhythmias. The compressible air causes obstruction to right ventricular ejection at the level of the pulmonary outflow tract. This particularly occurs following a bolus air embolism. Slower infusions of air become trapped at the level of the pulmonary arterioles, causing pulmonary hypertension and subsequent right ventricular failure. More gradual air entrapment results in micro-emboli entering the circulation. These not only obstruct flow, but neutrophils, fibrin, red blood cells, fat globules and platelets build up around the bubble. The resulting ultrastructural damage leads to increased basement membrane permeability and pulmonary oedema.
* A change in heart sounds ('mill wheel' murmur) is a very late sign.
* Central venous pressure (CVP) is elevated in 25% of patients and pulmonary artery pressure (PAP) rises in 50%.

- Arterial blood gases may reveal hypoxaemia and, less commonly, hypercarbia.
- Doppler (if available) is exceedingly sensitive.

Differential diagnosis

- If *respiratory symptoms* predominate, consider pulmonary embolism, pneumothorax, bronchospasm and pulmonary oedema.
- If *cardiovascular signs* predominate, consider cardiogenic shock, hypovolaemia, myocardial failure and septic shock.

Treatment

Immediate resuscitative measures should be initiated following the principles of 'ABC'.

If blood pressure is normal:

1. The surgeon should squeeze the wound to prevent further air entry and/or flood the operative site with normal saline.
2. Occlude veins proximal to the site of entry.
3. Lower the operative site below the level of the heart.
4. Institute intravenous volume loading to elevate venous pressure.
5. Increase intrathoracic pressure with a Valsalva manoevre, thus reducing venous return.
6. If possible, express bubbles through the wound.
   If during laparoscopy, **cease insufflation**.
7. Give 100% oxygen. **Stop nitrous oxide**. Nitrous oxide is 34 times more soluble than nitrogen and will diffuse rapidly into the bubble, increasing its size. Administering 100% oxygen will increase the partial pressure of oxygen in the blood and tissues, favouring nitrogen diffusion out of bubbles and into alveoli, leading to nitrogen washout.

If blood pressure is reduced:

As above, plus:
- Cardiopulmonary resuscitation may be required.
- If a CVP line is *in situ*, try to aspirate air from the right atrium. The optimum site for the CVP catheter tip is in the right atrium 2 cm below the junction with the superior vena cava.
- Place the patient in the left lateral decubitus position to overcome the airlock within the right ventricle by positioning it superior to the right ventricular outflow.
- Inotropic agents will increase cardiac contractility and may help improve cardiac output and systemic blood pressure, overcoming increased pulmonary vascular resistance.

- With massive air embolism, air can be removed from the pulmonary artery at thoracotomy or the patient can be placed on cardiopulmonary bypass as a last resort.

Further reading

Muth CM, Shank ES. Primary care: gas embolism. *N Engl J Med* 2000; **342**:476–82.

Palmon SC, Laurel EM, Lundberg J, Toung T. Venous air embolism: a review. *J Clin Anesth* 1997; **9**:251–7.

Porter JM, Pidgeon C, Cunningham AJ. The sitting position in neurosurgery: a critical appraisal. *Br J Anaesth* 1999; **82**:117–28.

2 Alarming cyanosis

> Describe the management of a patient with central cyanosis.

Actions

1. Check the pulse – if absent, treat for cardiac arrest.
2. Check gas flow settings on rotameters.
3. Immediately increase F_IO_2 and decrease vaporiser setting.
4. Monitor ECG, S_aO_2, $ETCO_2$.

Ventilation

Controlled ventilation

Does chest move normally?

If not, *attempt manual inflation using reservoir bag and breathing circuit.*

- Lungs easy to inflate – fault in ventilator, gas supply or breathing system.
- Lungs impossible or difficult to inflate:
  - (a) Check endotracheal tube (ETT):
  - ? misplaced in the oesophagus or pharynx (check $ETCO_2$)
  - ? blocked, kinked (inspect with laryngoscope and pass stout catheter through the tube to check patency)
  - ? herniated cuff (check pharynx dry, then deflate cuff)
  - ? bronchial intubation (withdraw tube slightly)
  - (b) Check chest: see FAULT IN CHEST.

If the chest moves normally, there is a fault in:
- chest – see FAULT IN CHEST
- circulation – see FAULT IN CIRCULATION
- oxygen source – see FAULT IN OXYGEN SUPPLY.

Spontaneous ventilation

- *Breathing appears obstructed.* Fault may be in:
  - airway – if not intubated, check pharynx and larynx are clear and intubate if necessary; if intubated, check ET tube
  - chest – see FAULT IN CHEST.
- *Breathing appears normal.* Fault may be in:
  - chest – see FAULT IN CHEST
  - circulation – see FAULT IN CIRCULATION
  - oxygen source – see FAULT IN OXYGEN SUPPLY.
- *Respiratory minute volume seems inadequate.* Intubate and ventilate, if necessary. Treat common causes:

- excessive volatile agent
- excessive narcotic agent
- muscle relaxant still active.

Fault in chest

- *Bronchospasm* – listen for wheeze.
  - **Note that severe bronchospasm may be silent**.
- *Fluid in alveoli* – listen for crackles and wheezing, check for (pink) frothy sputum.
- *Pneumothorax* – absent breath sounds over upper chest with hyper-resonant percussion note (may be bilateral).
- *Haemothorax or pleural effusion* – absent breath sounds over dependent part of lung.

Fault in circulation

There is a weak pulse:
- venous return reduced
- severe heart failure
- massive pulmonary embolism
- severe adverse drug reaction.

Fault in oxygen supply

- Source exhausted.
- Machine leaking (measure F_IO_2 with oxygen meter on inspiratory limb of breathing system).
- Pipeline cross-connection (check with F_IO_2 meter, change to cylinder supply if in any doubt).
- Breathing system:
  - fresh gas supply inadequate
  - leak
  - incorrect assembly.

Miscellaneous causes (rare)

- Malignant hyperpyrexia.
- Methaemoglobinaemia – consider if patient on sodium nitroprusside, GTN, prilocaine, sulphonamides. Give methylene blue 1 mg/kg.

Sometimes the cause is not obvious. If in doubt:
- change ETT
- ventilate with expired air as temporary measure
- change anaesthetic machine
- use gas cylinders.

Remember the common causes of cyanosis:
- misplaced ETT
- disconnection
- obstruction in breathing circuit
- oxygen supply failure
- cardiac arrest.

Capnography and oxygen meters are vital aids in diagnosis.

3 Bloody epidural

> Describe the management of an epidural catheter aspirating fresh blood shortly after placement.

- *Bleeding via Tuohy needle* – abandon attempt and try a different space (preferably above).
- *Bleeding via catheter:*
  - Slight – withdraw catheter by 1–2 cm (**not** through needle), flush with 10 mL of sterile isotonic saline and wait 2–3 minutes. If no further bleeding on aspiration, proceed with epidural.
  - **Use test dose.**
  - Frank – withdraw catheter and attempt a different space (preferably above).

Further reading

Brown DL. Spinal, epidural and caudal anaesthesia. In: Miller RD (ed.) *Anaesthesia*. Edinburgh: Churchill Livingstone, 1994, pp. 1505–34.

4 Dural tap

> Describe the management of accidental dural puncture in obstetrics.

Diagnosis

There is leakage of cerebrospinal fluid (CSF) through a Tuohy needle or catheter. The incidence of accidental dural puncture varies from 0.2% to 4%. The most common adverse event reported after accidental dural puncture is postdural puncture headache (PDPH), with a reported incidence of 60–90%.

Puncture of the dura with a Tuohy needle usually results in obvious flow of CSF through the needle. CSF tests positive for glucose on a reagent strip.

Actions

1. Withdraw the Tuohy needle.
2. Insert an epidural catheter using a different space (preferably above).
   Observe effects of test dose of local anaesthetic very carefully.
3. In obstetric cases, further labour needs careful management with discussion between anaesthetist, patient, midwife and obstetrician. Prolonged pushing should be avoided, but instrumental delivery is not always inevitable.
4. At the end of the procedure leave the epidural catheter (with Millipore filter) *in situ*. Administration of fluid into the epidural space acts as an obstructive pressure gradient against the leakage of CSF from the subarachnoid space. Fluid can be administered as intermittent bolus doses or continuous infusion. Prophylactic administration of 60 mL of preservative-free saline has been shown to reduce the severity of headache associated with accidental dural puncture. Pain on injection of the bolus should be taken as an immediate indication to stop, as it may indicate high pressure around the nerve roots. The second method of administering saline is under gravity feed into the epidural space. Infusions of volumes greater than one litre have not been shown to improve outcome compared to larger volumes.
5. The patient should lie flat for 24 hours.
6. Ensure high fluid intake – IV or oral (4 litres per 24 hours).
7. Follow-up the patient.

8. Consider an autologous blood patch if symptoms persist beyond 2–3 days. Blood administered into the epidural space forms a clot over the defect in the dural membrane so preventing further leakage. Inject 5–20 mL of blood slowly over 2–3 minutes via the Tuohy needle or epidural catheter, into the epidural space. The patient should lie still for several hours after the procedure and avoid excessive straining or heavy lifting in the following week. This reduces the risk of the patch being forced off the dura. History of previous epidural blood patch is not a contraindication to subsequent central neurological blockade.

   Immediate blood patch is not recommended.

Further reading

Berger CW, Crosby ET, Grodecki W. North American survey of the management of dural puncture occurring during labour epidural analgesia. *Can J Anaesth* 1998; **45**:110–4.

Carrie LES. Postdural puncture headache and extradural blood patch. *Br J Anaesthesia* 1993; **71**:179–80 (editorial).

Gleeson CM, Reynolds F. Accidental dural puncture rates in UK obstetric practice. *Int J Obstet Anesth* 1998; **7**:242–6.

5 Malignant hyperpyrexia

Describe the management of malignant hyperthermia.

Malignant hyperthermia is an inherited disorder of skeletal muscle that can be pharmacologically triggered to produce a combination of hypermetabolism, muscle rigidity and muscle breakdown. The incidence of reported malignant hyperthermia reactions varies from $1:40\,000$ to $1:100\,000$ anaesthetics. Estimates of the population prevalence of the genetic susceptibility are between $1:5000$ and $1:10\,000$.

The diagnosis of malignant hyperthermia may not be obvious at first. The primary features of malignant hyperthermia are a direct consequence of loss of skeletal muscle cell calcium homeostasis with a resulting increased intracellular calcium ion concentration. Some or all of the following signs may be present. If suspicious, insert a temperature probe immediately.

Signs

- There is a high and rising end-tidal CO_2.
- S_pO_2 falls as oxygen delivery is incapable of meeting the metabolic demands of stimulated muscle. Skeletal muscle constitutes 40% of body mass.
- Muscle rigidity (especially trismus) is due to continuous actin–myosin interaction:
  - either following suxamethonium ($\pm$ fasciculation)
  - or during the course of anaesthesia.
- There is a rapid rise in body temperature: 1°C every ten minutes.
- There may be sudden onset of unexplained tachycardia.
- Tachypnoea is a feature.
- Cardiac arrhythmias are due to hyperkalaemia secondary to rhabdomyolysis.
- Blood pressure is unstable.
- There may be unexplained cyanosis.
- Disseminated intravascular coagulation may occur as a result of the release of tissue clotting activators from muscle and through the resulting hyperthermia.
- Blood analysis – decreasing P_aO_2, increasing P_aCO_2, decreasing pH, decreasing (HCO_3), increasing plasma K^+ concentration. Plasma myoglobin concentrations are sufficient to cause renal tubular damage and acute renal failure.

Treatment

1. **Abandon the procedure or terminate surgery as soon as possible.**
2. **Stop inhalational agents.** Maintain anaesthesia with intravenous drugs whilst surgery is concluded.
3. Give 100% oxygen. If possible, hyperventilate with 2–3 times predicted minute volume. *Vecuronium or atracurium may be used to facilitate ventilation but may not overcome muscle spasm.*
4. Active cooling measures should be commenced, including infusion of cold intravenous solutions, application of ice in the axillae and groins and a cooling mattress.
5. Give dantrolene by rapid intravenous infusion. Dantrolene is the only drug effective in limiting the accumulation of calcium ions within muscle cells. Dantrolene 20 mg is presented with mannitol 3 g which is required to solubilise the dantrolene. Repeated doses of dantrolene (20 mg in adults, 1 mg/kg in children under 20 kg) should be administered until pyrexia, tachycardia and rise in end-tidal CO_2 subside. Repeat as necessary to a total of 10 mg/kg (average requirement is 3 mg/kg). Avoid using calcium-channel blocking drugs as they can produce marked cardiac depression when used in combination with dantrolene.
6. Give a large dose of glucocorticoid (e.g. methylprednisolone 2 g) to the average adult.
7. Acidosis is treated with bicarbonate and hyperkalaemia with insulin and dextrose. Treatment is guided by regular blood gases and electrolyte measurements.
8. A diuresis of at least 2 mL/kg per hour should be maintained to limit renal tubular damage by myoglobin.
9. Correct raised K^+ with 50 mL of 50% dextrose with 10 units of soluble insulin.
10. If dysrhythmias are present, follow the advanced life support (ALS) arrhythmia algorithm.
11. Inotrope to maintain cardiac output.
12. When the patient is adequately rehydrated (as assessed by CVP and haemotocrit) maintain adequate urinary output (>1 mL/kg per hour) with diuretic if necessary.
13. Body temperature may be unstable for 24–48 hours.
14. After the acute episode check for hypokalaemia, myoglobinuria and disseminated intravascular coagulation (DIC).
15. Admit to ICU.

Notes
* Each vial of dantrolene contains 20 g dantrolene sodium and 3 g mannitol, and requires 60 mL of water to reconstitute (pH 9.5).
* If the episode has been controlled and surgery is essential, use a 'safe' technique:
    * regional block with local anaesthetic (plain bupivacaine)
    * thiopentone, propofol, fentanyl, vecuronium, atracurium and pancuronium are all considered 'safe'
    * follow-up patients and family.

Further reading
Halsall PJ, Ellis FR. Malignant hyperthermia. *Anaesth Intens Care Med* 2002; 3:222–5.

Hopkins PM, Ellis FR. *Hyperthermic and Hypermetabolic Disorders*. Cambridge: Cambridge University Press, 1996.

Hopkins PM, Halsall PJ, Ellis FR. Diagnosing malignant hyperthermia susceptibility. *Anaesthesia* 1994; **49**:373–75 (editorial).

Kaplan RF. Malignant hyperthermia. In: *American Society of Anesthesiologists' Annual Refresher Course Lectures*, vol. 552, 1993, pp. 1–7.

Urwyler A, Deufel T, McCarthy TV, West SP for the EMHG. Guidelines for the molecular testing of susceptibility to malignant hyperthermia. *Br J Anaesth* 2001; **86**:283–7.

6 Pulmonary aspiration

> Describe the management of pulmonary aspiration in the anaesthetised patient.

The incidence of pulmonary aspiration syndrome is reported as 0.01%. It is more common with coughing during direct laryngoscopy and emergency surgery despite cricoid pressure. Sixty-three per cent of patients who aspirate are asymptomatic. It is thought that a volume of aspirate of at least 0.8 mL/kg is required to cause pulmonary aspiration syndrome.

Signs

Signs to look out for are:

*   cyanosis
*   coughing
*   tachypnoea
*   bronchospasm
*   possible hypotension and/or fever (usually late signs).

Actions

1. Place the patient in a head-down position and on side.
2. Start laryngoscopy and suction (consider bronchoscopy if solid matter inhaled).
3. Deliver 100% oxygen.

If the patient is paralysed:

1. Proceed with tracheal intubation.
2. Apply suction via an ETT in the head-down position. (Test aspirate with pH paper. If acid, this confirms gastric aspiration.)
3. Institute intermittent positive-pressure ventilation (IPPV) with at least 50% O_2, plus positive end-expiratory pressure (PEEP) if required.
4. If bronchospasm develops, treat with salbutamol 250 µg IV or aminophylline 250 mg IV.
5. As necessary:
    blood gas analysis
    colloid for hypotension.
6. Proceed with surgery if essential and if the patient's condition permits.
7. Pass a nasogastric tube and aspirate the stomach.
8. Obtain a chest x-ray.
9. Start chest physiotherapy.

If the patient is not paralysed:

1. Allow the person to wake up.
2. Apply high inspired oxygen concentration by facemask.
3. If bronchospasm develops, treat with nebulised salbutamol (2.5 mg). If this is inadequate use salbutamol 250 µg IV or aminophylline 250 mg IV.
4. As necessary:
    blood gas analysis
    colloid for hypotension.
5. If surgery is essential, consider a regional technique. If general anaesthesia is indicated:
    Pass nasogastric tube and aspirate stomach. Give 30 mL sodium citrate.
    Pre-oxygenate. Induce anaesthesia and intubate using cricoid pressure.
6. Obtain chest x-ray.
7. Start chest physiotherapy.

Further management

If there is clinical evidence of aspiration the patient will require observation in ICU (or possibly HDU) and possibly elective IPPV. All require postoperative O_2. It is generally thought that antibiotic treatment should be directed at proven infection, rather than given prophylactically. Steroids are no longer recommended.

Postpartum, reflux may persist for up to 48 hours despite gastric pH and volume of stomach contents returning to normal values within about 6–8 hours.

Further reading

Bogod DG. The postpartum stomach: when is it safe? *Anaesthesia* 1994; **49**:1 2.

Mendelson CL. The aspiration of stomach contents into the lungs during obstetric anaesthesia. *J Obst Gynaecol* 1946; **52**:191.

7 Severe drug reactions

> Describe the management of a severe drug reaction.

Diagnosis

There will be:
- flushing and urticaria
- hypotension
- bronchospasm.

Treatment

1. **Stop all suspected drugs.**
2. Stop or curtail surgery if possible.
3. For any severe reactions, adrenaline is the drug of choice. Use 100 µg boluses; i.e. 1 mL of 1:10000 adrenaline IV (1 mg made up to 10 mL total with normal saline). Titrate according to response.
4. For hypotension:
   Elevate legs.
   Give oxygen.
   Fluid: 2 litres of fluid (ideally colloid) over 10 minutes may be required.
   Establish ECG monitoring; consider CVP and arterial monitoring in severe reactions.
   Consider adrenaline infusion (5 mg in 500 mL saline, at 10–85 mL per hour) or other appropriate inotropic support if hypotension is prolonged.
5. Bronchospasm:
   Give oxygen.
   Give bronchodilator (e.g. nebulized salbutamol 2.5–5 mg or IV salbutamol 250 µg or aminophylline 250 mg).
   Ventilate if exhausted.
   Check arterial blood gases to ensure adequate ventilation.
6. With gross flushing and urticaria, consider an antihistamine (e.g. chlorpheniramine (Piriton) 10–20 mg IV).
7. Use of steroids is debatable in the acute phase, but may help reduce late deterioration.
8. Patients must be closely monitored for at least 6 hours after the event for coagulopathies (APTT, PT, fibrinogen, FBC), renal function (urine output, U&E), cardiovascular and respiratory adequacy.
9. *Inform the patient of the drug responsible and clearly record details in the notes.*

Establish cause

Collect blood samples: 5 mL in EDTA tube as soon as possible, then further samples at 3, 6 and 24 hours. Send the samples to the pathology laboratory to spin off the plasma and store at −20°C. Also, send samples taken at 10 min, 20 min, 1 hour and 24 hours after the event to haematology for WBC (total and differential), platelets and Hb.

Further reading

Association of Anaesthetists. *Anaphylactic Reactions Associated with Anaesthesia*. London: Association of Anaesthetists, 1993.

Hunter JM. Histamine release and neuromuscular blocking drugs. *Anaesthesia* 1993; **48**:561–3 (editorial).

Watkins J. Investigations of allergic and hypersensitivity reactions to anaesthetic agents. *Br J Anaesthesia* 1987; **59**:104–11.

8 Systemic toxicity of local anaesthetics

Describe the management of systemic toxicity due to local anaesthetics.

Symptoms and signs

- 1. Signs awake include:
  - tinnitus
  - light-headedness
  - visual disturbances
  - circumoral numbness
  - slurred speech
  - fine twitching of small muscles of the face and hands
  - drowsiness.
  - These early symptoms are related to the rich blood and nerve supply of the tongue, mouth and face. They usually occur at blood lignocaine levels of $\geq 2\,\mu g/mL$ and blood bupivacaine levels of $\geq 1.5\,\mu g/mL$.
- Drowsiness occurs in some patients.
- Convulsions may be triggered by the limbic system causing seizures that electrographically resemble temporal lobe epilepsy. This occurs at blood lignocaine levels $> 12\,\mu g/mL$, and blood bupivacaine levels $> 4\,\mu g/mL$.
- There may be apnoea and hypotension.
- Other signs are: increased P–R interval, AV dissociation, prolonged QRS, sinus bradycardia leading to asystole. Bupivacaine is also associated with ventricular arrhythmias, tachycardia and fibrillation. Bupivacaine is highly protein-bound to myocardial tissue.

Actions

ABC

1. Maintain airway and give 100% oxygen.
2. Intubate and ventilate if appropriate.
3. Treat convulsions: increments of IV thiopentone 50 mg, or diazepam 2.5 mg.
4. For hypotension (rare if no hypoxia):
     ephedrine 5 mg increments IV
     elevate legs
     IV fluids.
5. For cardiac arrest: the antiarrhythmic of choice for local anaesthetic induced ventricular arrhythmias is bretylium 400–700 mg IV.

Commence DC shock at 360 J and persist with CPR.

Further reading

Advanced Life Support Working Party of the European Resuscitation Council. Guidelines for advanced life support. *Resuscitation* 1992; **2**:111–22.

Tucker GT. Local anaesthetic drugs: mode of action and pharmacokinetics. In: Nimmo WS, Rowbotham DJ, Smith G (eds) *Anaesthesia*, 2nd edn. Oxford: Blackwell Scientific, 1994, pp. 1355–87.

9 Tricyclic overdose

> Outline the clinical features of an overdose of a tricyclic antidepressant.

The patient may initially be asymptomatic for 2–3 hours as absorption occurs. Tricyclic antidepressants inhibit reuptake of noradrenaline at nerve terminals, potentiating the action of adrenaline, noradrenaline and other catecholamines.

Signs

CNS features
- Agitation → seizures → coma.
- Anticholinergic features of the drug will cause pupils to be enlarged through this.

Cardiovascular features
These are secondary to quinidine-like membrane stabilizing effects.
- ↑ in catecholamines at autonomic synapses.
- Anticholinergic effects.
- Tachycardia → PR prolongation → QT prolongation → QRS prolongation.
- Hypertension → CV collapse.
- Proceeds to any of:
  - right bundle branch block (RBBB)
  - second- or third-degree heart block
  - VF/VT/asystole.

The tricyclics have a very high degree of protein binding and they bind avidly to myocardial tissue, causing the above effects. The degree of binding to myocardium and the clinical features vary with pH:
- Alkalosis leads to reduced binding to myocardium and reduction in CVS effects.
- IV bicarbonate will result in improvement in clinical features.

10 Wheezing

Describe the management of wheezing under anaesthesia.

Causes

- *Equipment:*
  - endotracheal tube inserted too far
  - kinked or partially blocked tube
  - over-inflated endotracheal tube cuff.
- *Patient:*
  - bronchial asthma (especially if inadequately anaesthetised)
  - pulmonary oedema.
- *Drugs:*
  - histamine-releasing drugs
  - non-selective beta-blockers
  - adverse drug reaction.

A wheeze throughout the respiratory cycle suggests obstruction within the equipment.

Actions

ABC. Call for senior help.
1. Relieve equipment cause.
2. Increase F_IO_2.
3. Monitor ECG.
4. Bronchodilators:
   Nebulised salbutamol 2.5–5 mg, or 250 µg IV.
   Aminophylline 250–500 mg IV slowly, followed by infusion of 0.5 mg/kg per hour.
   Consider deepening anaesthesia or changing inhalation agent to halothane if available.
   In life-threatening bronchospasm, adrenaline should be considered. Use 100 µg IV increments.
5. Hydrocortisone 100 mg IV 4-hourly.
6. Paralyse and ventilate if the patient is exhausted, if $P_aCO_2 > 8$ kPa (60 mmHg), and with increasing heart rate or falling blood pressure.
7. Check chest x-ray to rule out pneumothorax, pulmonary oedema, aspiration or other pathology when the patient is stable.

Further reading

Cottam S, Eason J. The intensive care management of acute asthma. In: Kaufman L (ed.) *Anaesthesia Review*, vol. 8. London: Churchill Livingstone, 1991, pp. 71–88.

McFadden ER. Fatal and near-fatal asthma. *N Engl J Med* 1991; **324**:409–10.

Peterfreund RA. Pathophysiology and treatment of asthma. *Curr Opin Anaesthesiol* 1994; **7**:284–92.

Multiple-choice questions: Action plans

1. In the early detection of an air embolism, the following are useful:
   a) ECG
   b) ultrasound
   c) end-tidal CO_2
   d) fall in blood pressure
   e) change in ventilatory pattern.

2. High central venous pressure, low blood pressure and acute circulatory failure are found in:
   a) tension pneumothorax
   b) pulmonary embolism
   c) congestive cardiac failure
   d) venous air embolism
   e) haemorrhage.

3. In acute cardiac tamponade there is:
   a) ascites
   b) hypotension
   c) bradycardia
   d) a prominent 'a' wave in the CVP trace
   e) cyanosis and cold extremities.

4. Immediate treatment of venous air embolism during posterior fossa surgery should include the following:
   a) turn the patient right side down
   b) give mannitol
   c) raise the intracranial venous pressure
   d) give a rapid fluid infusion
   e) turn off nitrous oxide.

5. Recognised features of fat embolism include:
   a) mental confusion
   b) bradycardia
   c) petechial rash
   d) respiratory distess syndrome
   e) pyrexia.

6. In cardiopulmonary resuscitation:
   a) lignocaine should be given before adrenaline in ventricular fibrillation
   b) the optimal treatment of ventricular tachycardia involves synchronised 50-joule DC shock
   c) the tracheal dose of adrenaline is 0.5 mg
   d) 50 mL $NaHCO_3$ should be given every 10 minutes
   e) calcium should be given to renal failure patients on dialysis.

7. Hypokalaemia
   a) causes ST segment depression on the ECG
   b) causes mental depression
   c) precipitates digoxin toxicity
   d) may precipitate muscle paralysis
   e) occurs in untreated hyperosmolar non-ketotic diabetic coma.

8. After massive inhalation of gastric acid one would expect the following:
   a) lung abscess
   b) severe hypercapnia
   c) bacteraemia
   d) hypovolaemia
   e) destruction of surfactant.

9. Postoperative hypoxia at 15 minutes may be due to:
   a) mild hypercapnia
   b) nitrous oxide diffusion
   c) central depression
   d) increased V/Q scatter
   e) shivering.

10. Ventricular arrhythmias are more common in the presence of:
   a) hypokalaemia
   b) hypoxia
   c) thyrotoxicosis
   d) cardiopulmonary bypass and digoxin treatment
   e) essential hypertension.

11. Treatment of acute anaphylaxis includes:
   a) IM adrenaline
   b) H_1 and H_2 antagonists
   c) hydrocortisone
   d) IM chlorpromazine
   e) IV salbutamol.

12. Air embolus is signified by:
  a) ECG changes
  b) Doppler ultrasound
  c) pulsus paradoxus
  d) raised CVP
  e) decreased end-tidal CO_2.

13. The following can be given by inhalation without causing systemic effects:
  a) adrenaline
  b) orciprenaline
  c) isoprenaline
  d) beclomethasone
  e) sodium cromoglycate.

14. Complications of dextran-70 include:
  a) hypocoagulability
  b) interference with cross-matching
  c) hypervolaemia
  d) renal failure
  e) antigenic reaction.

15. Recognised causes of urinary retention include:
  a) ketamine
  b) morphine
  c) amitriptyline
  d) ephedrine
  e) frusemide.

16. In epiglottitis the following are true:
  a) IV access and oxygen are essential first-line treatment
  b) immediate lateral neck x-ray is needed to aid diagnosis
  c) IV chlorpromazine is the treatment of choice
  d) tracheostomy should be performed if the patient is still intubated after 72 hours
  e) patient is likely to be intubated for 5 days.

17. Causes of prolonged postoperative recovery of consciousness are:
  a) acromegaly
  b) intraoperative intracerebral event
  c) myxoedema
  d) prolonged action of muscle relaxants
  e) hypoventilation.

18. TURP syndrome:
   a) is associated with hypokalaemia
   b) may present with convulsions
   c) is prevented by spinal anaesthesia
   d) is caused by blood loss
   e) requires treatment with diuretics.
19. A young man admitted to casualty following a road traffic accident is found to have central dislocation of the hip and is shocked. Likely causes are:
   a) ruptured bladder
   b) ruptured urethra
   c) blood loss
   d) neurogenic shock
   e) fat embolism.
20. A patient with vomiting, respiratory distress, cyanosis, epigastric tenderness and subcutaneous emphysema in the neck may be suffering from:
   a) ruptured oesophagus
   b) ruptured diaphragm
   c) ruptured trachea
   d) spontaneous pneumothorax
   e) pulmonary embolus.
21. Cricoid pressure:
   a) is effective in the presence of a nasogastric tube
   b) requires a complete cricoid cartilage to be effective
   c) should be performed with the neck extended
   d) should be performed after 5 minutes of pre-oxygenation
   e) compresses the oesophagus against the cervical vertebrae.

Answers to multiple-choice questions

1.	a) False;	b) True;	c) True;	d) False;	e) False
2.	a) True;	b) True;	c) True;	d) True;	e) False
3.	a) False;	b) True;	c) False;	d) True;	e) True
4.	a) False;	b) False;	c) True;	d) True;	e) True
5.	a) True;	b) False;	c) True;	d) True;	e) True
6.	a) False;	b) False;	c) False;	d) False;	e) True
7.	a) True;	b) False;	c) True;	d) True;	e) True
8.	a) False;	b) False;	c) False;	d) True;	e) True
9.	a) True;	b) False;	c) True;	d) True;	e) True
10.	a) True;	b) True;	c) True;	d) True;	e) True
11.	a) True;	b) True;	c) True;	d) False;	e) True
12.	a) True;	b) True;	c) False;	d) True;	e) True
13.	a) False;	b) False;	c) False;	d) True;	e) True
14.	a) True;	b) True;	c) True;	d) False;	e) True
15.	a) False;	b) True;	c) True;	d) True;	e) True
16.	a) False;	b) False;	c) False;	d) False;	e) False
17.	a) True;	b) True;	c) True;	d) True;	e) True
18.	a) False;	b) True;	c) False;	d) False;	e) True
19.	a) False;	b) False;	c) True;	d) False;	e) False
20.	a) True;	b) True;	c) True;	d) False;	e) False
21.	a) False;	b) True;	c) True;	d) False;	e) True

SECTION TWO

ANATOMY

1 First rib

Give an account of the anatomy of the first rib.

The first rib is the key to the important neurovascular relationships of this region. It is unique in being the shortest, flattest and most curvaceous of the ribs. Its extreme flattening and curvature gives it broad upper and lower surfaces and sharp outer and inner margins, the latter bearing the scalene tubercle or the tubercle of Lisfranc.

The 1st rib and the 1st thoracic vertebra form the thoracic inlet which is kidney-shaped because of the forward projection into it of the body of the 1st thoracic vertebra. It measures some 10 cm in diameter and 3 cm anteroposteriorly.

The inlet slopes downwards sharply from behind forwards, forming an angle of about 60 degrees with the horizontal. There is a 4-cm difference between the anterior and posterior extremities of the inlet, the upper border of the manubrium lying between the 2nd and 3rd thoracic vertebrae. During forced inspiration and expiration, the upper border of the manubrium moves about the length of a vertebral body in each direction.

The 1st rib has a head, with a single facet for the body of the 1st thoracic vertebra, a long neck and prominent tubercle, which articulates with the transverse process of the 1st thoracic vertebra.

Crossing the neck medially are the:
* sympathetic trunk
* superior intercostal artery with accompanying vein
* large branch of the anterior ramus of the 1st thoracic nerve passing to the brachial plexus.

The scalene tubercle provides the insertion for the tendon of scalenus anterior. Immediately in front of this tubercle, the upper surface of the rib bears a groove for the subclavian vein; because of the obliquity of the thoracic inlet this vessel lies well below and safely behind the clavicle. Behind the scalene tubercle lies a second groove which is for the subclavian artery and the lower trunk (C8, T1) of the brachial plexus. The groove is particularly well marked when the patient has a 'post-fixed' brachial plexus with a large contribution from T2. Immediately behind this groove is the area of insertion of scalenus medius.

Thus, anterior to the tubercle are:
1. Scalenus medius insertion
2. Subclavian artery
3. Subclavian artery groove
   Lower trunk (C8, T1) of brachial plexus.
   Well-marked groove when post-fixed brachial plexus with large contribution from T2.

4. Scalene tubercle – insertion for tendon of scalenus anterior
5. Groove for subclavian vein
6. Subclavious muscle – anterior extremity of the upper surface of the rib to become inserted in the under aspect of the clavicle

> *Inner margin of ribs:*
> To the inner margin of the 1st rib is attached the suprapleural membrane, better known as Sibson's fascia. This is a tough sheet of fibrous tissue which spreads out like a tent from its origin, the transverse process of C7, to form a protective covering of the cervical pleura.

7. Sematus anterior on lateral aspect of margin of 1st rib
8. Intercostal muscles
9. Cervical pleura – inferior aspect.

Relationships

Superior

Posterior to anterior:
1. Sympathetic trunk
2. Superior intercostal artery and vein
3. Large branch of the anterior ramus of the 1st thoracic nerve passing to the brachial plexus

- Prominent tubercle

4. Scalenus medius insertion
5. Subclavian artery
6. Subclavian artery groove

> Lower trunk of brachial plexus (C8, T1).
> Well-marked groove if post-fixed brachial plexus with large contribution from T2.

- Scalene tubercle – insertion for scalenus anterior tendon

7. Groove for subclavian vein
8. Subclavius muscle – anterior extremity of upper surface of the rib to become inserted in the under aspect of the clavicle. Usually able to prevent fragments of a comminuted fracture of the clavicle from piercing the sub-clavian artery.

Inferior

Lies against cervical pleura.

Lateral aspect

1. Attachment of scalenus anterior
2. Attachment of intercostal muscles.

Medial aspect

The inner margin is attached to the suprapleural membrane, better known as Sibson's fascia. This is a tough sheet of fibrous tissue which spreads out like a tent from its origin, the transverse process of C7, to form a protective covering over the cervical pleura.

2 Anterior spinal artery

> Describe the anatomy of the anterior spinal artery. Discuss its clinical significance.

The anterior spinal artery is a midline vessel lying on the anterior median fissure and is formed at the foramen magnum by the union of a branch from each vertebral artery supplying the whole of the cord in front of the posterior grey columns.

Origin

The anterior spinal artery arises above from branches of the vertebral arteries and descends in front of the anterior longitudinal sulcus of the spinal cord. It receives contributions from the spinal arteries which reach the spinal cord by way of the intervertebral foramina and enter the extradural space to reach spinal nerve roots in the region of the dural cuffs.

Branches

The spinal arteries receive collateral blood flow along their course:
1. Branches of the vertebral artery
2. Multiple segments of the intercostal and lumbar arteries
3. Internal iliac arteries
4. Artery of Adamkiewicz, or greater radicular artery, which usually enters unilaterally on the left (in 78%), by way of a single intervertebral foramen, between T8 and L3. In a small number of patients, the artery of Adamkiewicz enters at a higher level, T5. Iliac tributaries are then larger.

In all, six or seven vessels feed the anterior spinal artery.

Termination

The anterior spinal artery terminates where the spinal cord terminates, namely at level L2.

Clinical significance

Anterior spinal artery ischaemia causes a predominantly motor lesion, as the anterior two-thirds of the cord, including the anterior horn cells, are supplied exclusively by this artery.

Spinal cord ischaemia may occur if a feeding spinal artery is traumatised by a needle inserted towards a spinal nerve root. The artery of Adamkiewicz is the major feeder entering via a single invertebral foramen between T8 and L3. Damage to this artery may result in ischaemia of the lumbar enlargement of the cord.

Paraplegia is an uncommon but devastating consequence of thoracic, thoracoabdominal or even abdominal reconstructive surgery. Spinal cord damage may follow translumbar abdominal aortography during the surgical intervention. There is a 0.25% incidence of spinal cord damage following aortic surgery. Incidence of spinal cord damage is 10 times more prevalent in ruptured compared to unruptured aneurysms. The most common neurological deficits are complete flaccid paraplegia with disassociated sensory loss. The expected incidence of lower-limb neurological effects varies according to the extent and cause of the aneurysm.

Spinal cord ischaemia and paraplegia following thoracoabdominal aortic aneurysm repair have been attributed variously to increased cerebrospinal fluid (CSF) pressure associated with hypertension proximal to the cross-clamp, the site and duration of cross-clamp application, intraoperative hypertension, and accidental permanent interruption of critical lower intercostal and lumbar arteries.

Attempts to limit the incidence of cord injury have included hypothermia (now largely abandoned), proximal–distal aortic shunting, and careful preservation of large intercostal arteries. The administration of barbiturates may reduce spinal cord oxygen consumption, perhaps thereby helping to preserve neurological function.

3   Blood supply of the heart

Describe the anatomy of the blood supply and venous drainage of the heart.

Arterial blood supply

The arterial blood supply to the cardiac musculature is derived from the right and left coronary arteries.

The *right coronary artery* (RCA) arises from the anterior sinus and passes forwards between the pulmonary trunk and right atrium. It descends in the right part of the atrioventricular groove. At the inferior border of the heart it continues along the atrioventricular groove to anastomose with the left coronary artery at the inferior interventricular groove. It gives off a marginal branch along the lower border of the heart and an interventricular branch which runs forward in the inferior interventricular groove to anastomose near the apex of the heart with the corresponding branch of the left coronary artery. The RCA supplies the:

- lateral wall of the right ventricle
- posterior wall of the right ventricle
- inferior wall of the left ventricle
- sinoatrial node in 55% of patients.

In 85% of patients the RCA terminates as the posterior descending artery – right dominant.

The left coronary artery is larger than the right. It arises from the aortic sinus. It passes first behind and then to the left of the pulmonary trunk, reaches the left part of the atrioventricular groove in which it runs laterally round the left border of the heart to reach the inferior interventricular groove.

The left coronary artery divides into the left anterior descending (LAD) artery and circumflex artery. The LAD artery gives rise to the diagonal branches. It supplies:

- the anterolateral wall of the left ventricle
- the interventricular septum
- the anterior wall of the right ventricle
- the ventricular apex.

The circumflex artery gives rise to the obtuse marginal arteries. Together they supply the:

- left atrium
- posterior wall of the left ventricle
- lateral wall of the left ventricle.

Venous drainage of the heart

About two-thirds of the venous drainage of the heart is by veins which accompany the coronary arteries and which open into the right atrium. The rest of the blood drains by means of small veins (venae cordis minimae) directly into the cardiac cavity.

The coronary sinus lies in the posterior atrioventricular groove and opens into the right atrium just to the left of the mouth of the inferior vena cava.

The coronary sinus receives the:

- great cardiac vein in the anterior interventricular groove
- middle cardiac vein in the inferior interventricular groove
- small cardiac vein which accompanies the marginal artery along the lower border of the heart
- oblique vein which descends obliquely on the back of the left atrium and which opens near the left extremity of the coronary sinus.

The anterior cardiac vein lies in the anterior atrioventicular groove. It drains much of the anterior surface of the heart and opens directly into the right atrium.

4 Femoral nerve

Describe the anatomy of the femoral nerve. How would you perform a femoral nerve block?

Femoral nerve of the thigh

The femoral nerve emerges from nerve roots L2, L3 and L4. It is the largest nerve of the lumbar plexus and supplies the muscles and the skin of the anterior compartment of the thigh.

The nerve emerges from the lateral margin of psoas, passes downwards in the groove between psoas and iliacus to both of which it sends a nerve supply, then enters the thigh beneath the inguinal ligament.

Relationships

At the base of the femoral triangle the nerve lies on iliacus, a finger's breadth lateral to the femoral artery, from which vessel it is separated by a portion of psoas.

The femoral triangle is a triangular area situated in the upper part of the medial aspect of the thigh. It is bounded superiorly by the inguinal ligament, laterally by the sartorius, and medially by the medial border of the adductor longus muscle. Its floor is gutter-shaped and formed from lateral to medial by the ilio-psoas, the pectineus and the adductor longus. The skin and fascia of the thigh form its roof.

The femoral triangle contains the terminal part of the femoral nerve and its branches, the femoral sheath, the femoral artery and its branches, the femoral vein and its tributaries, and the deep inguinal lymph nodes.

Branches of the femoral nerve

Almost at once within the femoral triangle the nerve breaks up into its terminal branches which stem from an anterior and posterior division.
* *Anterior division*
  * Muscular branches to – pectineus and sartorius.
  * Cutaneous branches to – intermediate and medial cutaneous nerves of thigh.
* *Posterior division*
  * Muscular branches to – quadriceps.
  * Cutaneous branch to – saphenous nerve.
  * Articular branches – to hip and knee.

Anterior division

Muscular branches

The nerve to pectineus passes behind the femoral sheath, in which is contained the femoral artery and vein, and enters the anterior surface of pectineus. This muscle receives, in addition, an inconsistent supply from the accessory obturator nerve.

The nerve to sartorius arises either from, or in common with, the intermediate cutaneous nerve of the thigh, and enters the medial aspect of sartorius in its upper third.

Cutaneous branches

The intermediate cutaneous nerve of the thigh divides into two branches, which supply the front of the thigh down to the knee.

The medial cutaneous nerve of the thigh passes medially across the femoral vessels, then divides into anterior and posterior branches. The anterior branch pierces the deep fascia at the lower third of the thigh to supply the skin over the medial side of the lower thigh as far as the knee. Here the nerve links up with the patellar plexus. The posterior branch runs along the border of sartorius, supplying twigs to the overlying skin and communicating with the obturator and saphenous nerves. At the knee, the nerve pierces the deep fascia and supplies an area of skin over the medial side of the leg; an area which is inversely proportional to the contribution from the obturator nerve. Thus the lateral, intermediate and medial cutaneous nerves penetrate the deep fascia in echelon, roughly along the oblique line formed by sartorius.

Posterior division

Muscular branches

The nerve to rectus femoris enters the deep aspect of the muscle near its origin. Rectus femoris is the only part of the quadriceps to act on the hip as well as the knee, and its nerve is the only part of the quadriceps nerve supply to give a branch to the hip joint (Hilton's law – the same trunks of nerves whose branches supply the groups of muscles moving a joint, furnish also a distribution of nerves to the skin over the insertions of the same muscles, and the interior of the joint receives its nerves from the same source.) The nerve to vastus intermedius may be bifid or trifid and enters the front of its muscle.

The nerve to vastus lateralis reaches its muscle by passing deep to rectus femoris in company with the descending branch of the lateral circumflex femoral branch of the profunda femoris artery.

All three nerves to the vasti send filaments of supply to the knee.

Cutaneous branches

The saphenous nerve is the largest cutaneous branch of the femoral nerve and the only cutaneous branch to originate from the posterior division. It arises in the femoral triangle, descends lateral to the artery, and then enters the adductor canal of Hunter, where it crosses in front of the artery to lie on its medial side. The nerve escapes from the lower part of the canal by emerging between sartorius and gracilis, runs down the medial border of the tibia immediately behind the saphenous vein, crosses with the vein in front of the medial malleolus and reaches as far as the base of the great toe, supplying an extensive cutaneous area over the medial side to the knee, leg, ankle and foot.

Immediately on leaving the adductor canal, the saphenous nerve gives off its intrapatellar branch, which pierces sartorius and is distributed to the skin immediately below the knee as part of the patellar plexus. This branch is sometimes divided by the incision for a medial menisectomy.

With regard to the arterial branches to hip and knee, if the femoral nerve is damaged there is loss of knee extension due to quadriceps paralysis and anaesthesia over the front of the thigh. Overlap from other cutaneous nerves usually prevents sensory loss on the medial side of the leg and foot.

The femoral nerve block

The patient should lie in the supine position with the hip slightly abducted and externally rotated. The anterior superior iliac spine and pubic tubercle are identified. A line joining these two structures overlies the inguinal ligament. The femoral artery is identified and the point where it emerges from beneath the inguinal ligament is marked.

Femoral nerve block is accomplished by placing the index finger at the lateral side of the femoral artery to 'guard' it. The point of insertion is 2 cm lateral to the point where the artery emerges from beneath the inguinal ligament. A 22-gauge needle is used. It first pierces fascia lata, which is usually 1.5–3 cm deep in a normal-sized adult, then the fascia iliaca approximately 0.5 cm deeper. Passing through each fascial layer is usually perceived as a 'pop'.

Once the needle tip has passed through the fascia iliaca, the solution may then be injected as a bolus, or infiltrated as a fan across the path of the nerve. A peripheral nerve stimulator should elicit a twitch of quadriceps muscles (not the sartorius muscle). However, at this point in its course the femoral nerve may have divided into a number of branches, which slide away from the needle easily.

'Three-in-one' block

This is an alternative to the discrete femoral nerve block. As the femoral, lateral cutaneous and obturator nerves are formed within psoas, they are enclosed within a fascial sheath, which continues to encase the nerves on their journey to the periphery. Placing a sufficient volume of injectate within this sheath and encouraging its proximal spread to the lumbar plexus or nerve roots results in a high incidence of block of all three nerves.

A 6- to 8-cm 22-gauge needle is inserted as for a femoral nerve block but at an angle of 45 degrees to the horizontal, aiming the tip of the needle to the manubrium sterni. The position of the needle is adjusted to obtain an appreciable twitch of the quadriceps with a peripheral nerve stimulator (PNS). At this point, the tip of the needle lies under the inguinal ligament and in the centre of the nerve. By moving the needle from medial to lateral, twitches of the vastus medialis and lateralis, respectively, may be obtained as the needle sweeps across the nerve.

A twitch of sartorius muscle may be very misleading and should not be interpreted as a quadriceps twitch, as the sartorius is very superficial to the femoral nerve.

The position of the tip of the needle should be adjusted so that a twitch of the quadriceps and the patella is obtained at a stimulation intensity of 0.4–0.6 mA. To prevent distal spread of the injectate, the sheath distal to the point of injection should be occluded digitally, and occlusion maintained for 5 minutes after injection of 30 mL of solution. This technique results in proximal spread of injectate to the plexus, and even root level, with a high incidence of block of all three major branches of the lumbar plexus.

5 Internal jugular veins

Give an account of the anatomy of the internal jugular veins.

The internal jugular vein receives blood from the brain, face and neck. The vein has a dilatation at its upper end, the superior bulb, and another near its termination, the inferior bulb. Directly above the inferior bulb is the cuspid valve.

Origin

The internal jugular vein runs from its origin at the jugular foramen in the skull where it continues in the sigmoid sinus, to its termination behind the sternal extremity of the clavicle where it joins the subclavian vein to form the brachiocephalic (innominate) vein.

Course

It lies lateral first to the internal, and then to the common carotid artery within the carotid sheath. In its upper part the vein lies quite superficially in the anterior triangle of the neck, superficial to the external carotid artery. It then descends deep to sternomastoid.

Relationships

- *Anterolaterally:* the skin, superficial fascia, platysma, transverse cutaneous nerve, investing layer of deep cervical fascia, sternocleidomastoid, parotid salivary gland. Its lower part is covered by the sternothyroid, sternohyoid and omohyoid muscles, which intervene between the vein and the sternocleidomastoid. The ansa cervicalis crosses the vein. Higher up, it is crossed by the stylohyoid, the posterior belly of digastric, the posterior auricular and occipital arteries, and the accessory nerve. The styloid process and the stylopharyngeus muscles separate the vein from the parotid gland. The chain of deep cervical lymph nodes runs alongside the vein.
- *Posteriorly:* the transverse processes of the cervical vertebrae, levator scapulae, scalenus medius, scalenus anterior, cervical plexus, phrenic nerve, thyrocervical trunk, vertebral vein, the first part of the subclavian artery. On the left it passes in front of the thoracic duct.
- *Medially:* above, the internal carotid artery and the 9th, 10th, 11th and 12th cranial nerves; below, the common carotid artery and the vagus nerve.

Tributaries

- *Inferior petrosel sinus.* This assists in draining the cavernous sinus. It leaves the skull through the anterior part of the jugular foramen and joins the internal jugular vein at or below the superior bulb.

- *Facial vein.* Having left the face and crossed superficially over the submandibular salivary gland, it is joined by the anterior division of the retromandibular vein. The vein then crosses the hypoglossal nerve, the loop of the lingual artery, and the external and internal carotid arteries to join the internal jugular vein.
- *Pharyngeal veins.* These drain the pharyngeal venous plexus and join the facial, lingual, or internal jugular vein.
- *Lingual vein.* This joins the facial vein or drains into the internal jugular vein.
- *Superior thyroid vein.* This leaves the superior pole of the thyroid gland and drains into the facial or internal jugular vein.
- *Middle thyroid vein.* This leaves the lobe of the thyroid gland and drains into the internal jugular vein at the level of the cricoid cartilage.
- *Occipital vein.* This occasionally accompanies the occipital artery and drains into the internal jugular vein. More often it joins the vertebral or posterior auricular veins.

6 Oesophagus

Describe the anatomy of the oesophagus.

The oesophagus has its origin at the laryngopharynx at the level of C6. It is a tubular structure about 25 cm long which is continuous above with the laryngeal part of the pharynx opposite C6. It passes through the diaphragm at the level of T10 to join the stomach, and conveys masticated enteral nutrients from the mouth to the rest of the gastrointestinal (GI) tract. It terminates at the stomach 1.3 cm below the diaphragm.

Course and relationships

1. *Neck:* In the neck it lies in front of the vertebral column. Laterally, it is related to the lobes of the thyroid gland, and anteriorly it is in contact with the trachea and the recurrent laryngeal nerves.
2. *Thorax:* The oesophagus passes downward and to the left through the superior and then posterior mediastinum. At the level of the sternal angle the aortic arch pushes the oesophagus over to the midline.

The *relationships of the thoracic oesophagus* are:

- *Anteriorly:* Trachea and left recurrent laryngeal nerve; the left main bronchus, which constricts it, and the pericardium which separates the oesophagus from the left atrium.
- *Posteriorly:* Bodies of the thoracic vertebrae, the thoracic duct, the azygous veins, and the right posterior intercostal arteries and, at the lower end, the descending thoracic aorta.
- *Right side:* Mediastinal pleura and the terminal part of the azygous vein.
- *Left side:* Left subclavian artery, the aortic arch, the thoracic duct and the mediastinal pleura.
- *Inferiorly:* To the level of the roots of the lungs, the vagus nerves leave the pulmonary plexus and join the sympathetic nerves to form the oesophageal plexus. The left vagus lies anterior to the oesophagus and the right vagus posterior.

At the opening in the diaphragm the oesophagus is accompanied by the two vagi, branches of the left gastric blood vessels and lymphatic vessels.

Fibres from the right crus of the diaphragm pass around the oesophagus in the form of a sling.

In the abdomen the oesophagus is related to the left lobe of the liver anteriorly and to the left crus of the diaphragm posteriorly.

Supply and drainage

Blood supply

The upper third of the oesophagus is supplied by the inferior thyroid artery, the middle third by branches from the descending thoracic aorta, and the lower third by branches from the left gastric artery.

The veins from the upper third drain into the inferior thyroid veins, the middle third into the azygous veins, and the lower third into the left gastric vein, a tributary of the portal vein.

Lymphatic drainage

Lymph vessels from the upper third of the oesophagus drain into the deep cervical nodes, from the middle third into the superior and posterior mediastinal nodes, and from the lower third into the nodes along the left gastric blood vessels and the coeliac nodes.

Nerve supply

The oesophagus is supplied by the parasympathetic and sympathetic afferent and efferent fibres via the vagi and sympathetic trunks. In the lower part of its thoracic course, the oesophageal nerve plexus surrounds the oesophagus.

7 Subclavian vein

Describe the anatomy of the right subclavian vein. What are the complications of the technique of subclavian cannulation?

The right subclavian vein is the continuation of the axillary vein. It runs from the lateral border of the 1st rib, arches over the rib in the groove in front of the insertion of scalenus anterior to join the internal jugular vein behind the sternoclavicular joint.

Relationships

- *Superior.* The vein is most cephalad at the level of the midpoint of the clavicle. Overlying the vein is firstly the clavicle and then medially fascia and skin.
- *Lateral.* Laterally it lies anteroinferiorly to the subclavian artery as it crosses the 1st rib. At the medial side of the 1st rib, scalenus anterior separates the vein from the artery.
- *Posterior.* The subclavian vein crosses in front of the phrenic nerve and costotransverse fascia (Sibson's) overlying the pleura.
- *Anterior.* The external jugular vein joins the subclavian vein after passing through the deep fascia above the clavicle.

Complications of subclavian vein cannulation

Pneumothorax
Haemothorax
Hydrothorax
Subcutaneous emphysema
Brachial plexus palsy
Phrenic nerve palsy
Phrenic nerve paralysis

Subclavian artery puncture
Innominate vein puncture
Subclavian vein thrombosis
Knotted catheter
Air embolism
Infection

8 Diaphragm

Describe the anatomy of the diaphragm.

The diaphragm constitutes the great muscular septum between the thorax and the abdomen. It is one of the distinguishing features in mammalian anatomy.

The diaphragm consists of peripheral muscle with a central tendon of strong interlacing bundles blending above with the fibrous pericardium.

Origin

It arises from the crura, the arcuate ligaments, the costal margin and xiphoid:
- The crura arises from the lumbar vertebral bodies – the left from L1 and L2, the right from L1, L2 and L3.
- The arcuate ligaments are the:
  - *median* – a fibrous arch joining the two crurae
  - *medial* – a thickening of the fascia over psoas
  - *lateral* – a condensation of fascia over quadratus lumborum ending laterally near the tip of the 12th rib.
- The costal origin is from the tips of the last six costal cartilages.
- The xiphoid origin comprises two slips from the posterior aspect of the xiphoid.

Diaphragmatic foramina

There are three major openings:
- level of T8 – inferior vena cava
- level of T10 – the oesophagus, together with the vagus and oesophageal vessels
- level of T12 – the aorta together with the thoracic duct and azygos vein, behind the median arcuate ligament at T12.
  There are additional openings:
- The sympathetic trunk passes behind the medial arcuate ligament.
- The splanchnic nerves pierce the crura.
- The hemiazygous vein drains through the left crus.
- Superior epigastric vessels pass between the xiphoid and costal origins of the diaphragm into the posterior rectus sheath.
- The lower intercostal nerves and vessels enter the anterior abdominal wall between the interdigitations of diaphragm and transversus abdominus.
- Lymphatics stream from the retroperitoreal tissues through the diaphragm to the mediastinum.

The oesophageal hiatus is reinforced by a sling of muscle fibres from the right crus. This probably plays a part in maintaining competence at the oesophagogastric junction.

Nerve supply

1. The phrenic nerve (C3, C4 and C5) provides the motor supply of the diaphragm, apart from an unimportant contribution to the crura from T11 and T12.
2. Section of the phrenic nerve is followed by complete atrophy of the corresponding hemidiaphragm.
3. Proprioceptive fibres from the centre of the diaphragm are transmitted via the phrenic nerve.
4. The periphery of this muscle has its sensory supply from the lower thoracic nerves.
5. The right phrenic nerve pierces the central tendon to the lateral side of the inferior vena cava. The left phrenic nerve pierces the muscle about 1 cm lateral to the attachment of the pericardium.

9 Pleura

> Give an account of the anatomy of the pleura.

The pleurae consist of double-walled serous-lined sacs, one in each hemithorax. They have a visceral layer which invests the lung itself and passes onto its fissures, and a parietal layer, which clothes the diaphragm, the chest wall, the apex of the thorax and the mediastinum.

Origin and termination

The two layers meet at the site of invagination which is the lung root or hilum. Here the pleura hangs down as a fold, rather like an empty sleeve, termed the pulmonary ligament. Between the two layers of the pleura is a potential space, the pleural cavity which is moistened with a film of serous fluid, permitting the two lengths to move on each other with the minimum of friction.

Embryology: During the development of the lungs, each lung bud invaginates the wall of the coelomic cavity and then grows to fill the greater part of that cavity. Thus the lung becomes covered with visceral pleura and the thoracic wall with parietal pleura. The original coelomic cavity is reduced to a slit-like space called the pleural cavity as the result of the lung growth.

Course and relationships

The parietal layer lines the thoracic wall, covers the thoracic surface of the diaphragm and the lateral aspect of the mediastinum, and extends into the root of the neck to line the undersurface of the suprapleural membrane at the thoracic inlet.

The visceral layer completely covers the outer surfaces of the lungs and extends into the depths of the interlobular fissures. For the purposes of description, it is customary to divide the parietal pleura according to the regions in which it lies or the surface that it covers:

- *Cervical pleura*. This extends up into the neck, lining the undersurface of the supra pleural membrane. It reaches a level about 2–3 cm above the medial third of the clavicle.
- *Costal pleura*. This lines the inner surfaces of the ribs, the costal cartilages, the intercostal spaces, the sides of the vertebral bodies, and the back of the sternum.
- *Diaphragmatic pleura*. This covers the thoracic surface of the diaphragm. In quiet respiration the costal and diaphragmatic pleurae are in opposition to each other below the lower border of the lung. In deep inspiration the margins of the base of the lung descend, and the costal and diaphragmatic pleurae separate. This lower area of the pleural cavity into which the lung

expands on inspiration is referred to as the costodiaphragmatic recess. The recess is 5 cm deep in the scapula line posteriorly, 9 cm in the midaxillary line and 4 cm in the midclavicular line.

- *Mediastinal pleura.* This covers and forms the lateral boundary of the mediastinum. At the root of the lung it is reflected as a cuff around the vessels and bronchi and here becomes continuous with the visceral pleura.

Nerve supply

The parietal pleura is supplied as follows:
1. The costal pleura is segmentally supplied by the intercostal nerves.
2. The mediastinal pleura is supplied by the phrenic nerve.
3. The diaphragmatic pleura is supplied over the domes by the phrenic nerve and around the periphery by the lower five intercostal nerves.
4. The visceral pleura covering the lungs receives an autonomic vasomotor supply, but is insensitive to common sensations such as pain and touch.

Lines of pleural reflection

The pleural margins can be mapped out on the chest wall as follows:
1. The apex of the pleura extends about 3 cm above the midpoint of the clavicle. The margin then passes behind the sternoclavicular joint and meets the opposite pleural edge behind the sternum at the 2nd costal cartilage level.
2. At the 4th costal cartilage, the left pleura deflects to the lateral margin of the sternum, corresponding to the cardiac notch of the underlying lung, and then descends to the 6th costal cartilage.
3. The right pleural edge continues vertically downwards and projects a little below the right costoxiphoid angle.
4. The pleural lower margin lies at the level of the 8th rib in the midclavicular line, and the 10th rib at the mid-axillary line which is its lowest level. It terminates behind at the level of the spine of the 12th thoracic vertebrae, descending posteriorly slightly below the costal margin at the costovertebral angle.

10 Arterial supply of brain

Outline the arterial supply of the brain and its meninges.

The brain and spinal cord are surrounded by three membranes or meninges: the dura mater, arachnoid mater and pia mater.

Dural arterial supply

Numerous arteries supply the dura mater from the internal carotid, maxillary, ascending pharyngeal, occipital and vertebral arteries. From the clinical standpoint, the most important is the middle meningeal artery, which is commonly damaged in head injuries.

The *middle meningeal supply* arises from the maxillar artery in the infratemporal fossa. It enters the skull through the forearm spinosum and runs forward and laterally in a groove on the upper surface of the squamous part of the temporal bone. It lies between the meningeal and endosteal layers of the dura. After a short distance the artery divides into anterior and posterior branches. The anterior branch passes forward and upward to the anterior inferior angle of the parietal bone. Here, the bone is deeply grooved by the artery for a short distance before it runs backwards and upwards on the parietal bone. The posterior branch passes backwards and upwards across the squamous part of the temporal bone to reach the parietal bone. The course of the arterial branch corresponds roughly to the line of the underlying precentral gyrus of the brain. The posterior branch curves backwards and supplies the posterior part of the dura mater.

Blood supply of the brain

The brain is supplied by the two internal carotid and the two vertebral arteries. The four arteries anastomose on the inferior surface of the brain and form the circulus arteriosus.

Internal carotid artery

This artery emerges from the cavernous sinus on the medial side of the anterior clinoid process by perforating the dura mater. It then enters the subarachnoid space by piercing the arachnoid mater and turns backwards to the region of the anterior perforated substance of the brain, at the medial end of the lateral cerebral sulcus. Here it divides into the anterior and middle cerebral arteries.

The following are branches of the cerebral portion of the internal carotid artery:

- *Ophthalmic artery*. This arises as the internal carotid artery emerges from the cavernous sinus. It enters the orbit through the optic canal, below and lateral to the optic nerve.
- *Posterior communicating artery*. This runs posteriorly to join the posterior cerebral artery.
- *Choroidal artery*. A small branch, it passes backwards, enters the inferior horn of the lateral vehicle, and ends in the choroid plexus.
- *Anterior cerebral artery*. This runs anteriorly and medially and enters the longitudinal fissure of the cerebrum. It is joined to the fellow on the opposite side by the anterior communicating artery. It curves posteriorly over the corpus callosum, and its cortical branches supply all the medial surface of the cerebral cortex as far back as the parieto-occipital sulcus. The branches also supply a strip of cortex about 2.5 cm wide on the adjoining lateral surface. The anterior cerebral artery thus supplies the 'leg area' of the precentral gyrus. A number of central branches pierce the brain substance and supply the deep masses of grey matter within the cerebral hemisphere.
- *Middle cerebral artery*. The largest branch of the internal carotid, it runs laterally in the lateral cerebral sulcus. Cortical branches supply the entire lateral surface of the hemisphere, except for the narrow strip supplied by the anterior cerebral artery, the occipital pole, and the inferolateral surface of the hemisphere, which are supplied by the posterior cerebral artery. This artery thus supplies all the motor area except the 'leg area'. Central branches enter the anterior perforated substance and supply the deep masses of grey matter within the cerebral hemisphere.

Vertebral artery

The vertebral artery, a branch of the first part of the subclavian artery, ascends through the foramina in the transverse processes of the upper six cervical vertebrae. It enters the skull through the foramen magnum and passes upward, anteriorly and medially on the medulla oblongata. At the lower border of the pons it joins the vessel of the opposite side to form the basilar artery.

Cranial branches of the vertebral artery are:
- meningeal arteries
- anterior and posterior spinal arteries
- posterior inferior cerebellar artery
- medullary arteries.

Basilar artery

The basilar artery, formed by the union of the two vertebral arteries, ascends in a groove on the anterior surface of the pons. At the upper border of the pons it divides into the two posterior cerebral arteries.

The basilar artery gives off branches to:
- the pons, cerebellum and internal ear
- the posterior cerebral arteries.

The posterior cerebral artery on each side curves laterally and backward around the midbrain. Cortical branches supply the inferolateral surface of the temporal lobe and the lateral and medial surfaces of the occipital lobe. Central branches pierce the brain substance and supply the deep masses of grey matter within the cerebral hemisphere and the midbrain.

Circle of Willis

This lies in the interpeduncular fossa at the base of the brain. It is formed by the anastomosis between the two internal carotid arteries and the two vertebral arteries. The anterior communicating, the anterior cerebral, the internal carotid, the posterior communicating, the posterior cerebral and the basilar arteries all contribute to the circle. The circle of Willis (circulus arteriosus) allows blood that enters by either internal carotid or vertebral arteries to be distributed to any part of both cerebral hemispheres.

11 Brachial plexus

> Describe the anatomy of the brachial plexus and describe your technique for an axillary brachial plexus block.

The brachial plexus provides the motor innervation and nearly all the sensory supply of the upper limb.

Formation of the brachial plexus

The plexus is formed by the anterior primary rami of C5–T1. In addition there is frequently a contribution above from C4 and another below from T2.

Occasionally the plexus is mainly derived from C4–C8 (pre-fixed plexus) or from C6–T2 (post-fixed plexus), variations which are normally associated with the presence of a cervical rib or of an anomalous 1st rib respectively.

The five roots of the plexus emerge from the invertebral foramina. Each of those from C5, C6 and C7 passes behind the foramen transversarium of its respective cervical vertebra with its contained vertebral vessels, then lies in the gutter between the anterior and posterior tubercles of the corresponding transverse process. All five roots then become sandwiched between scalenus anterior and medius. Here the roots of C5 and C6 form the upper trunk, root C7 continues as the middle trunk, and those of C8 and T1 link into the lower trunk.

The three trunks emerge from between the scaleni and pass in a closely grouped cluster downward and laterally across the base of the posterior triangle and then across the 1st rib.

At the lateral border of the 1st rib, behind the clavicle, each trunk divides into an anterior and posterior division. The six divisions stream into the axilla and there join up into three cords: lateral, medial and posterior. These are named after the relationship they bear to the axillary artery.

Relationships

Roots

These are between the scalene muscles. The roots of the plexus lie *above* the *second part of the subclavian artery*.

Trunks

These are in the posterior triangle. The trunks of the plexus, *invested in a sheath of prevertebral fascia*, are superficially placed. They are covered only by skin, platysma and deep fascia. The trunks are, however, crossed by a number of structures:
- inferior belly of omohyoid
- external jugular vein

- transverse cervical artery
- supraclavicular nerves.

The upper and middle trunks lie above the subclavian artery as they stream across the 1st rib, but the *lower trunk lies behind the artery* and may groove the rib immediately posterior to the subclavian groove.

Divisions

At the *lateral border* of the 1st rib the trunks bifurcate into divisions which are *situated behind the clavicle*, the *subclavius muscle* and the *suprascapular vessels* and then descend into the axilla.

Cords

The cords are formed at the *apex* of the axilla, and become grouped around the axillary artery. At first the *medial cord lies behind the artery* with the *posterior and lateral cords lateral to this vessel*. Once behind pectoralis minor the cords take up their relations to the artery as signified by their names.

The interscalene sheath

As the roots of the brachial plexus emerge in the groove between the anterior and posterior tubercles of the transverse processes of the cervical vertebrae, they lie in a fibro-fatty space between two sheaths of fibrous tissue.

- The posterior part of the sheath arises from the posterior tubercles and covers the front of the middle scalene muscle.
- The anterior part of the sheath arises from the anterior tubercles and covers the posterior aspect of the anterior scalene muscle.

Laterally, the sheath extends as a covering around the brachial plexus as this emerges into the axilla. The significance of this space to the anaesthetist is that it forms a sheath around the brachial plexus into which local anaesthetic can be injected to produce a brachial plexus block.

Brachial plexus block: axillary perivascular technique

Full resuscitation equipment and monitoring in line with Association of Anaesthetists of Great Britain and Ireland guidelines should be available.

Axillary block is probably the most widely used technique of brachial plexus block. The area in which the block is carried out is far removed from (a) the dome of the lung, and (b) the phrenic nerve. Thus the likelihood of pulmonary complications is minimal.

The patient should be placed in the supine position with the arm abducted to approximately 90 degrees and the forearm flexed to 90 degrees and externally rotated so that the dorsum of the hand lies on the table and the forearm is parallel to the long axis of the patient's body. The patient's hand should not be behind his/her head as this position makes performance of the technique more difficult.

The final step in preparing to carry out an axillary block is to identify the axillary pulse. Hyperabduction of the arm will obliterate the axillary artery pulse in 83% of normal individuals. In very muscular individuals, if the degree of abduction of the arm is reduced to somewhat less than 90 degrees, identification of the arterial pulse is easier.

Performing the block

Having identified the axillary artery, the artery should be followed as far proximally as possible, ideally to the point where the pulse disappears under the pectoralis major muscle. If the needle can be inserted high enough in the axilla, the injection will be made above the level of the humeral head, which tends to obstruct the flow of anaesthetic solution injected below it.

With the index finger still on the pulse of the axillary artery, a short bevelled needle is inserted just superior to the finger tip, directing the needle towards the apex of the axilla so that the needle will be travelling in almost the same direction as the neurovascular bundle as it is advanced. When carrying out a right axillary block, palpation is best carried out with the index finger of the right hand, using the left hand to manipulate the needle.

The needle is advanced slowly, approaching the neurovascular bundle at a 10- to 20-degree angle until *one of three end-points* indicates that the tip of the needle lies in the perivascular sheath:

- *End-point 1.* A 'fascial click' will be felt if a short bevelled needle is used as the tip of the needle penetrates the *tough axillary sheath*. The cutting point needles do not give you this 'click'. Secondly, bevelled needles show a significant reduction in the incidence of neural damage.
- *End-point 2.* The needle is advanced slowly until a twitch is observed if using a peripheral nerve stimulator, or the patient reports paraesthesia in the distribution of one of the nerves that lies within the sheath at this level, indicating that the tip of the needle has encountered a nerve and hence lies in the axillary perivascular compartment.
- *End-point 3.* If bright red blood appears within the hub of the needle, the artery has been encountered and entered. When this occurs, the anaesthetist should **not** withdraw the needle but should advance it as quickly as possible through the posterior wall of the vessel, and inject the contents of the syringe. Some anaesthetists advocate the so-called 'transarterial technique'. They believe that penetration of the artery is the most certain and reproducible sign of entry into the axillary perivascular compartment.

When the axillary sheath has been penetrated, the tip of the needle should lie superiorly tangentially to the arterial wall, 20–40 mm proximal to the most proximal palpable point of pulsation and probably proximal to the humeral head. If properly placed, the needle will pulsate.

Local anaesthetic is injected. The actual volume depends on the patient's size, sex and age and the desired level of anaesthesia; 20–40 mL is the usual range. Throughout the injection repeated aspiration for blood should be carried out intermittently.

Firm digital pressure should be applied directly behind the needle during and immediately after the injection to prevent retrograde flow down the sheath.

When the injection of the appropriate volume of local anaesthetic has been completed, the needle is withdrawn until it lies in the subcutaneous tissue *directly over the artery*. At this point, 3–5 mL of local anaesthetic are deposited. This will effectively block the interostobronchial nerve and the medial brachial cutaneous nerve, if it lies outside the sheath.

As soon as the subcutaneous injection has been made, the needle should quickly be withdrawn and digital pressure maintained as the arm is brought down to the patient's side. This manoeuvre removes the obstruction to central flow provided by the humeral head when the arm is abducted.

Alternative methods
Other methods of brachial plexus block are:
- subclavian perivascular technique
- interscalene perivascular technique.

12 Innervation of the eye

> Describe the innervation of the eye. How may the anaesthetist affect intraocular pressure?

The orbit is a pyramidal-shaped bony cavity with an apex posteriorly and a base in front. It has a number of openings that transmit nerves and blood vessels from the brain. The nerve supply to the globe in the orbit and accessory structures is from the 2nd, 3rd, 4th, 5th, 6th and 7th cranial nerves.

Innervation of the eye

The *optic nerve* (2nd cranial) enters the orbit from the middle cranial fossa via the optic canal. Its length in the orbit is 3 cm, and sheaths of pia mater, arachnoid mater and dura mater surround it. It curves laterally and downwards as it passes forward within the muscle core of the eye, and pierces the sclera medial to the posterior pole of the globe, where the meninges merge with the sclera. The optic nerve receives the central retinal artery during its course. The nasociliary nerve, ophthalmic artery and superior ophthalmic vein lie on top of, and parallel to, the nerve. The short ciliary nerves and vessels surround the anterior portion of the nerve.

The *oculomotor nerve* (3rd cranial) divides into two branches before entering the orbit via the superior orbital fissure:

* The upper branch supplies the superior rectus and levator palpebrae superioris.
* The lower branch supplies the medial and inferior recti, inferior oblique and a motor root to the ciliary ganglion, which supplies the pupillary sphincter and ciliary muscle.

The *trochlear nerve* (4th cranial) and the *abducens nerve* (6th cranial) enter the orbit via the superior orbital fissure and supply the superior oblique and lateral rectus muscles respectively.

The *trigeminal nerve* (5th cranial) first division (opthalmic division) is entirely sensory. It is distributed to the eyeball, overlying conjunctiva, protective upper lid and adjacent lacrimal gland, the skin of the forehand, nose and scalp back as far as the vortex, the mucous membrane of the medial and lateral walls of the anterior part of the nose and to the adjacent frontal and ethmoidal sinuses.

The ophthalmic nerve passes along the lateral wall of the cavernous sinus, below cranial nerves III and IV, to reach the superior orbital fissure, where it divides into its lacrimal, frontal and nasociliary branches.

The *lacrimal nerve* is the smallest of the three branches and passes into the orbit through the lateral part of the superior orbital fissure above the fibrous ring of origin of the extrinsic orbital muscles. The lacrimal nerve emerges from the orbit below the lateral extremity of the orbital margin. Its terminal fibres supply the conjunctiva and a patch of skin of the upper lid adjacent to the outer canthus.

The *frontal nerve* is the largest branch of the opthalmic nerve. It passes through the superior orbital fissure above the orbital ring and above levator palpebrae superioris. Within the orbit it divides into the larger supra-orbital nerve and the smaller supratrochlear branch. The supratrochlear nerve passes above the pulley of the superior oblique muscle to supply the conjunctiva and the skin of the upper eyelid near the inner canthus.

The *nasociliary* nerve gives off a sensory contribution to the ciliary ganglion after entering through the orbital fissure. A second branch of this nerve divides into two *long ciliary nerves*, which enter the back of the eyeball and are sensory but also transmit sympathetic dilator pupillae fibres. A third branch of the nasociliary nerve, which innervates the eye, is the *infratrochlear nerve* innervating the conjunctiva near the inner canthus.

The *ciliary ganglion* is a parasympathetic ganglion situated on the lateral aspect of the optic nerve about 8 mm from the apex of the orbit. It receives three roots. A *sensory root* from the nasociliary nerve passes through the ganglion without synapsing and supplies the cornea, sclera, iris and ciliary body (but not the conjunctiva). A *parasympathetic root* (motor) consists of preganglianic fibres from the oculomotor (3rd) nerve. Postganglianic fibres leave the ganglion in the short ciliary nerves, which enter the globe. The *sympathetic root* (motor to the dilator pupillae and vasoconstrictor vessels of the eye) is derived from the superior cervical sympathetic ganglion via the internal carotid plexus. The fibres pass through the ciliary ganglion without synapsing.

Factors affecting intraocular pressure

Volume of contents of the globe

The balance between the production and drainage of *aqueous humor* is the primary physiological mechanism, which maintains intraocular pressure (IOP) at 16 ± 5 mmHg. Two-thirds of the aqueous is produced by active secretion from the ciliary process in the posterior chamber of the eye, utilising carbonic anhydrase and cytochrome oxidase. The remainder is formed by simple filtration through the anterior surface of the iris. The aqueous humor drains through the trabecular meshwork at the angle of the anterior chamber into the canal of Schlemm. From here the fluid enters the orbital venous system and hence to the internal and external jugular veins. Hence, avoiding increases in central venous pressure (CVP), from whatever cause, during anaesthesia is important to avoid direct transmission to the eye. Coughing can increase IOP to 35–40 mmHg transiently.

Choroidal blood flow is autoregulated, remaining constant over a wide range of mean perfusion pressures (90–130 mmHg). Below the lower limit, marked reductions in IOP occur; at systolic pressures of 50–60 mmHg it approaches zero. There is a linear increase in choroidal blood flow when P_aCO_2 increases from 4.5 to 9.1 kPa as the vessels are very sensitive to P_aCO_2. Respiratory alkalosis induced by mechanical ventilation induces choroidal vasoconstriction, thus lowering IOP. Hyperbaric oxygen is more vasoconstrictive to the choroid than hypocapnea, but this effect has not been used during eye surgery. Hypoxaemia should be avoided as this induces choroidal vasodilatation and elevates IOP.

Most of the blood from the choroid, ciliary body and iris enters the vortex veins, which perforate the sclera behind the equator to join the venous plexuses of the orbit. Any factor which results in venous engorgement of the head and neck causes an increase in IOP (coughing, vomiting, high inflation pressures and obstruction of the neck, veins by the tracheal tube tie).

Vitreous humor volume can be altered by the anaesthetist by administration of osmotic agents, which may be used to dehydrate the vitreous. Mannitol is effective but a maximum dose of 1.5 g/kg over 30–60 minutes should not be exceeded. Similarly sucrose 50% aqueous solution reduces IOP within 5 minutes. Its rapid action can be very useful if the ocular contents are bulging during surgery, but 1 g/kg should not be exceeded.

Extraocular compression of the globe

Extraocular compression by surgical retractors or anaesthetic facemasks must be avoided. Non-depolarising muscle relaxants help to reduce IOP by relaxing the extraocular muscles.

Suxamethonium has been demonstrated to cause a rise of 7–12 mmHg in IOP of rapid onset and 5–6 minutes' duration. The mechanism of action seems to be a rise in tone in the extrinsic muscles of the eye, but this has not been fully elucidated. Pre-curarisation may reduce, but does not abolish, the effects of suxamethonium on IOP. The intravenous administration, immediately prior to induction, of 500 mg of acetazolamide or of lignocaine has been shown to produce some suppression of the rise in IOP due to suxamethonium. Most intravenous induction agents, with the exception of ketamine, lower the IOP by reducing blood pressure. The subsequent administration of suxamethonium will cause the IOP to rise from its post-induction value, but this may not be higher than the pre-induction value.

Other anaesthetic factors

Premedication of patients who are apprehensive allows for a smoother induction and emergence, hence avoiding surges in blood pressure to a point. Benodiazepines are usually effective. The use of opioid analgesics, except in patients with pain, is best avoided as they increase the risk of vomiting, retching and ventilatory depression. Prophylactic antiemetics such as droperidol, prochlorperazine or metoclopramide may be of use.

Except for very minor extraocular procedures when a facemask can be used, all eye operations require a tracheal tube or laryngeal mask airway (LMA). Significantly smaller increases in IOP have been reported using the LMA, both on placement and removal, when compared to tracheal intubation. The LMA avoids difficult intubation and the need for suxamethonium.

13 Intercostal space

Describe the anatomy of the intercostal space.

The intercostal spaces are closed by thin but strong muscles and aponeuroses which course the nerves, blood vessels and lymphatics of the chest.

Intercostal muscles

The muscles of the intercostal spaces are disposed in three layers corresponding to the three layers of the lateral abdominal wall.

External intercostals
* *Origin* – outer border of the costal groove of the rib above.
* *Insertion* – directed downwards and forwards to the upper border of the rib below.
* *Extent* – from the superior costotransverse ligament posteriorly to the costochondral junction (from there to the sternum it is replaced by the external intercostal membrane).
* *Nerve supply* – corresponding intercostal nerves by collateral branches.
* *Action* – may elevate ribs during inspiration.

Internal intercostals
* *Origin* – floor of costal groove of rib above.
* *Insertion* – directed downwards and backwards to upper border of rib below.
* *Extent* – from side of sternum to angle of rib, then replaced to superior costotransverse ligament by the internal intercostal membrane.
* *Nerve supply* – corresponding intercostal nerves by collateral branches.
* *Action* – anteriorly, may raise ribs in inspiration; more posteriorly, may depress ribs in expiration.

Intercostals intimi
* *Origin* – medial border of the costal groove of the rib above.
* *Insertion* – may cross one or two ribs, blend with internal intercostal muscle at upper border of a rib.
* *Nerve supply* – corresponding intercostal nerves.
* *Action* – as internal intercostals (see above).

Sternocostalis
* *Origin* – deep aspect of xiphoid process, lower part of body of sternum and 5th, 6th and 7th costal cartilages.

- *Insertion* – radiate upwards and laterally to backs of 2nd to 6th costal cartilages.
- *Nerve supply* – intercostal nerves.
- *Action* – may raise xiphisternum (this has a weak inspiratory effect).

Subcostals

These are ill-defined slips extending over several ribs and lining the posterolateral part of the lower chest wall. They are supplied by intercostal nerves.

Levatores costarum

These are 11 small muscles, each arising from the tip of a thoracic transverse process and inserted into the upper border of the rib below, near the angle. The nerve supply is the dorsal rami of the corresponding intercostal nerves.

These four classes of muscle in the innermost layer are linked to each other by *membranous tissue* which is continuous superiorly with the suprapleural membrane (Sibon's fascia).

The neurovascular bundle

In each intercostal space lies a neurovascular bundle comprising (from above downwards):
- posterior intercostal vein
- posterior intercostal artery
- intercostal nerve.

This bundle is protected by the costal groove of the upper rib. Posteriorly, this bundle lies between the pleura and the posterior intercostal membrane. At the angle of the rib it passes between the internal intercostal and the intracostal muscles.

14 The axilla

> Describe the anatomy of the axilla.

The axilla, or armpit, is a pyramid-shaped space between the upper part of the arm and the side of the chest. The upper end or apex is directed into the root of the neck. It is bounded in front by the clavicle, behind by the border of the scapula, and medially by the outer border of the 1st rib. The lower end, or base, is bounded in front by the anterior axillary fold (formed by the lower border of the pectoralis major muscle), behind by the posterior axillary fold (formed by the tendon of latissimus dorsi and the teres major muscle) and medially by the chest wall.

Relationships

- *Anterior wall* – made by pectoralis major, subclavius, and pectoralis minor muscles, the clavipectoral fascia, and the suspensory ligament of the axilla.
- *Posterior wall* – by the subscapularis, latissimus dorsi and teres major muscles from above.
- *Medial wall* – by the upper four or five ribs and the intercostal space covered by the serratus anterior muscle.
- *Lateral wall* – by the coracobrachialis and biceps muscles in the bicipital groove of the humerus.
- *The base* – formed by the skin stretching between the anterior and posterior walls.

Contents of the axilla

Axillary artery

The artery begins at the lateral border of the 1st rib as a continuation of the subclavian artery and ends at the lower border of the teres major muscle, where it continues as the brachial artery. Throughout its course, the artery is closely related to the cords of the brachial plexus and their branches and is enclosed with them in a connective tissue sheath, called the axillary sheath. If this sheath is traced upwards into the root of the neck, it is seen to be continuous with the prevertebral fascia.

The pectoralis minor muscle passes in front of the axillary artery and, for the purposes of description, is said to divide it into three parts. The branches of the axillary artery supply the thoracic wall and shoulder region. The first part of the artery gives off one branch, the second part two branches and the third part three branches.

Axillary vein

The axillary vein is formed in the region of the lower border of the teres major muscle by the union of the venae comitantes of the brachial artery and the basilic vein. It runs upwards on the medial side of the axillary artery and ends at the lateral border of the first rib by becoming the subclavian vein.

The vein receives tributaries, which correspond to the branches of the axillary artery, and, in addition, it receives the cephalic vein.

Brachial plexus

The cords of the brachial plexus lie in the axilla. All three cords lie above and lateral to the first part of the axillary artery. The medial cord crosses behind the artery to reach the medial side of the second part of the artery. The posterior cord lies behind the second part of the artery and the lateral cord lies on the lateral side of the second part of the artery.

Branches of the brachial plexus

- *Nerve to subclavius.* Having descended in front of the trunks of the brachial plexus and the subclavian artery in the neck, it supplies the subclavian artery.
- *Long thoracic nerve.* This arises from the roots of the brachial plexus in the neck and enters the axilla by passing down over the lateral border of the 1st rib behind the axillary vessels and brachial plexus. It descends over the lateral surface of the serratus anterior muscle, which it supplies.
- *Lateral pectoral nerve.* This arises from the lateral cord of the brachial plexus. It pierces the clavipectoral fascia and supplies the pectoralis major muscle.
- *Musculocutaneous nerve.* This arises from the lateral cord of the brachial plexus. It supplies the coracobrachialis muscle and leaves the axilla by piercing that muscle.
- *Lateral root of the medial nerve.* This is the direct continuation of the lateral cord of the brachial plexus. It is joined by the medial root to form the median nerve trunk. This passes downward on the lateral side of the axillary artery. The median nerve gives off no branches in the axilla.
- *Medial pectoral nerve.* This arises from the medial cord of the brachial plexus. It supplies and pierces the pectoralis minor muscle, and supplies the pectoralis major muscle.
- *Medial cutaneous nerve of the arm.* This arises from the medial cord of the brachial plexus. It is joined by the intercostal brachial nerve. It supplies the skin on the medial side of the arm.
- *Medial cutaneous nerve of the forearm.* This arises from the medial cord and descends in front of the axillary artery.

- *Ulnar nerve.* This arises from the medial cord of the brachial plexus. It descends in the interval between the axillary artery and vein. The ulnar nerve gives off no branches in the axilla.
- *Medial root of the median nerve.* This arises from the medial cord of the brachial plexus. It crosses in front of the third part of the axillary artery to join the lateral root of the median nerve.
- *Upper and lower subscapular nerves.* These arise from the posterior cord of the brachial plexus. They supply the upper and lower parts of the subscapularis muscle.
- *Thoracodorsal nerve.* This arises from the posterior cord of the brachial plexus. It runs downward on the subscapularis to reach the latissimus dorsi muscle which it supplies. It accompanies the subscapular vessels.
- *Axillary nerve.* This is one of the terminal branches of the posterior cord of the brachial plexus. At the lower border of the subscapularis muscle, it turns backward and passes through the quadrilateral space in company with the posterior circumflex humeral artery. Having given off a branch to the shoulder joint, it divides into anterior and posterior branches.
- *Radial nerve.* This is a direct continuation of the posterior cord. It lies behind the axillary artery. It is the largest branch of the brachial plexus. Before leaving the axilla it gives off branches to the long and medial heads of triceps muscle and the posterior cutaneous nerve of the arm.

Lymph nodes

The axillary lymph nodes drain lymphatic vessels from the lateral part of the breast, the superficial lymphatic vessels from thoracoabdominal walls above the level of the umbilicus, and the vessels from the upper limb. The lymph nodes are arranged in six groups:
- *Anterior group.* Lying along the lower border of the pectoralis minor behind the pectoralis major, these nodes receive lymph vessels from the lateral part of the breast and superficial vessels from the anterolateral abdominal wall above the level of the umbilicus.
- *Posterior group.* Lying in front of the subscapularis muscle in association with the subscapular vessels, these nodes receive superficial lymph vessels from the back, down as far as the level of the iliac crests.
- *Lateral group.* Lying along the medial side of the axillary vein, these nodes receive most of the lymph vessels of the upper limb.
- *Central group.* Lying in the centre of the axilla in the axillary fat, these nodes receive lymph from the above three groups.
- *Infraclavicular group.* Lying in the clavipectoral fascia in the deltopectoral triangle, these nodes receive superficial lymph vessels from the lateral side of the hand, forearm and arm. The lymph vessels accompany the cephalic vein.

- *Apical group.* Lying at the apex of the axilla at the lateral border of the 1st rib, these nodes receive the efferent lymph vessels from all the other axillary nodes. The apical nodes drain into the subclavian lymph trunk. On the left side, this trunk drains into the thoracic duct; on the right side, it drains into the right lymphatic trunk. Alternatively, the lymph trunks may drain directly into one of the large veins at the root of the neck.

15 The sympathetic trunk

> Describe the anatomy of the sympathetic trunk.

The sympathetic trunk on each side is a ganglionated nerve chain which extends from the base of the skull to the coccyx, in close relationship to the vertebral column, maintaining a distance of about 2.5 cm from the midline throughout its course.

The cervical sympathetic trunk

The cervical part of the sympathetic trunk extends upwards to the base of the skull and below to the neck of the 1st rib where it becomes continuous with the thoracic part of the sympathetic trunk (see below). It lies directly behind the internal and common carotid arteries (i.e. medial to the vagus) and is embedded in deep fascia between the carotid sheath and the prevertebral layer of deep fascia.

The sympathetic trunk possesses three ganglia: the superior, middle and inferior cervical ganglia.

Superior cervical ganglion

This is a large ganglion which lies immediately below the skull. Branches are as follows:

* *Internal carotid nerve.* This consists of postganglion fibres, ascending from the upper pole of the ganglion. It accompanies the internal carotid artery into the carotid canal in the temporal bone. It divides into branches around the artery to form the internal carotid plexus.
* *Grey rami communicantes* – to the upper four anterior rami of the cervical nerves.
* *Anterior branches* – to the common and external carotid arteries. These branches form a plexus around the arteries and are distributed along the branches of the external carotid artery.
* *Cranial nerve branches.* These join the 9th, 10th and 12th cranial nerves.
* *Pharyngeal branches.* These unite within the pharyngeal branches of the glossopharyngeal and vagus nerves to form the pharyngeal plexus.
* *Superior cardiac branch.* This descends in the neck behind the common carotid artery. It ends in the cardiac plexus in the thorax.

Middle cervical ganglion

This is small and lies at the level of the cricoid cartilage. It is related to the loop of the inferior thyroid artery. Branches are as follows:

* *Grey rami communicantes* – to the anterior rami of the 5th and 6th cervical nerves.

- *Thyroid branches*. These pass along the inferior thyroid artery to the thyroid gland.
- *Middle cardiac branch*. This descends in the neck behind the common carotid artery. It ends in the cardiac plexus in the thorax.

Inferior cervical ganglion

The inferior cervical ganglion in the majority of subjects is fused with the first thoracic ganglion to form the stellate ganglion. It lies in the interval between the transverse process of the 7th cervical vertebra and the neck of the 1st rib, behind the vertebral artery. Branches are as follows:

- *Grey rami communicantes* – to the anterior rami of the 7th and 8th cervical nerves.
- *Arterial branches* – to the subclavian and vertebral arteries.
- *Inferior cardiac branch*. This descends behind the subclavian artery to join the cardiac plexus in the thorax.

The part of the sympathetic trunk connecting the middle cervical ganglion to the inferior or stellate ganglion is represented by two or more nerve bundles. The most anterior bundle crosses in front of the first part of the subclavian artery and then turns upwards behind it. The anterior bundle is referred to as the ansa subclavian.

The thoracic sympathetic trunk

The chain enters the thorax anterior to the neck of the 1st rib. It is continuous above with the cervical ganglion, and below with the lumbar parts of the sympathetic trunk. It is the most laterally placed structure in the mediastinum and runs downwards on the heads of the ribs. It leaves the thorax on the side of the body of the 12th thoracic vertebra by passing behind the medial arcuate ligament.

The thoracic sympathetic chain has 12 (often only 11) segmentally arranged ganglia, each with a white and grey ramus communicantes passing to the corresponding spinal nerve. The first ganglion is often fused with the inferior cervical ganglion to form the stellate ganglion.

Branches

- *Grey rami communicantes* go to all the thoracic spinal nerves. The postganglion fibres are distributed through the branches of the spinal nerves to the blood vessels, sweat glands and erector pili muscles of the skin.
- *The first five ganglia* give postganglionic fibres to the heart, aorta, lungs and oesophagus.
- *The lower seven ganglia* mainly give preganglionic fibres which are grouped together to form the splanchnic nerves and supply the abdominal viscera. They enter the abdomen by piercing the crura of the diaphragm.

- The greater splanchnic nerve arises from ganglia 5–9.
- The lesser splanchnic nerve arises from ganglia 10 and 11.
- The lowest splanchnic nerve arises from ganglion 12.

The thoracic sympathetic chain is covered, within the chest, by pleura and crosses in front of the intercostal vessels at each intervertebral space.

The abdominal sympathetic trunk

The abdominal part of the sympathetic trunk is continuous above with the thoracic and below with the pelvic parts of the sympathetic trunk. It runs downwards along the medial border of the psoas muscle on the bodies of the lumbar vertebrae. It enters the abdomen from behind the medial arcuate ligament and gains entrance to the pelvis below by passing behind the common iliac vessels. The right sympathetic trunk lies behind the right border of the inferior vena cava; the left sympathetic trunk lies close to the left border of the aorta.

The abdominal sympathetic trunk possesses four segmentally arranged ganglia, the first and second often being fused together. The upper two ganglia receive a white ramus communicans from the 1st and 2nd lumbar nerves.

Branches
- *Grey rami communicantes* – to the lumbar spinal nerves. The postganglionic fibres are distributed through the branches of the spinal nerves to the blood vessels, sweat glands and erector pili muscles of the skin.
- *Fibres pass medially* to the sympathetic plexuses on the abdominal aorta and its branches. These plexuses also receive fibres from splanchnic nerves and the vagus.
- *Fibres pass downward and medially* in front of the common iliac vessels into the pelvis, where, together with branches from the sympathetic nerves in front of the aorta, they form a large bundle of fibres called the hypogastric plexus.

The pelvic sympathetic trunk

The pelvic part of the sympathetic trunk is continuous above with the abdominal part. It runs down behind the rectum on the front of the sacrum, medial to the anterior sacral foramina. The sympathetic trunk has four or five segmentally arranged ganglia.

Branches
- *Grey rami communicantes* – to the sacral and coccygeal spinal nerves.
- *Fibres* that join the pelvic plexuses.

16 The trachea

> Describe the anatomy and histology of the trachea.

The trachea extends from its attachment at the *lower end of the cricoid cartilage*, at the level of C6, to its termination at the *bronchial bifurcation* at the level of T5 and the manubrio-sternal junction (angle of Louis). In full inspiration, the bronchial bifurcation can be at the level of T6.

In the adult the trachea is some 15 cm long, of which 5 cm lies above the suprasternal notch. This portion can be nearly 8 cm when the neck is fully extended.

The diameter of the trachea is correlated with the size of the subject. A good working rule is that it has the same diameter as the patient's index finger.

Patency of the trachea is due to a series of 16 to 20 C-shaped cartilages joined vertically by fibroelastic tissue and closed posteriorly by the unstriped *trachealis muscle*.

The cartilage of the tracheal bifurcation is the *heel-shaped carina*.

The trachea lies exactly in the mid-line in the cervical part of its course, but within the thorax it is deviated slightly to the right by the arch of the aorta.

Relationships in the neck

Arteriorly

The trachea is covered arteriorly by the skin and by superficial and deep fascia, through which the rings are easily felt. The second and fourth rings are covered by the isthmus of the thyroid, along whose upper border branches of the superior thyroid artery join from either side.

In the lower part of the neck the edges of the *sternohyoid and sternothyroid muscles* overlap the trachea, which is also covered by the *inferior thyroid veins*. The inferior thyroid veins stream downwards to the *innominate* (brachiocephalic) veins, by the cross-communication between the *arterior jugular veins* and, when present, by the *thyroidea ima artery*, which ascends from the arch of the aorta or from the brachiocephalic (innominate) artery.

It is because of this close relationship with the brachiocephalic artery that erosion of the tracheal wall by a tracheostomy tube may cause sudden profuse haemorrhage.

On each side are the lateral lobes of the thyroid gland, which intervene between the trachea and carotid sheath and its contents (common carotid artery, internal jugular vein and vagus nerve).

Posteriorly

The trachea rests on the oesophagus with the recurrent laryngeal nerves lying in a groove between the two.

Thoracic relationships

The trachea descends through the superior mediastinum.

Anteriorly

From above downwards lie the *inferior thyroid veins*, the *origins of the sterno-hyoid muscles* from the back of the manubrium, the *remains of the thymus*, the *brachiocephalic vein* (innominate) and, lastly, the arch of the aorta.

Posteriorly

As in its cervical course, the trachea lies throughout on the oesophagus, with the left recurrent laryngeal nerve placed in a groove between the left borders of these two structures.

The right and left sides

One the right side, the trachea is in contact with the mediastinal pleura, except where it is separated by the *azygos vein* and the *right vagus nerve*.

On the left side, the *left common carotid* and *left subclavian arteries*, the aortic arch and the left vagus intervene between the trachea and the pleura. The altering relationships between the major arteries and the trachea are due to the diverging, somewhat spiral, course of the arteries from their aortic origins to the root of the neck.

Supply

Blood supply

The arterial supply to the trachea is derived from the inferior thyroid arteries and the venous drainage is via the inferior thyroid veins. Lymphatics pass to the deep cervical, pretacheal and paratracheal nodes.

Nerve supply

The trachea is innervated by the laryngeal branch of the vagus nerve with a sympathetic supply from the middle cervical ganglion.

Histology of the trachea

The lining epithelium of the trachea and larger bronchi is in several layers:
* a basal layer which rests on a well-defined basal membrane
* an intermediate zone of spindle-shaped cells
* a superficial sheet of columnar ciliated cells which are interspersed with mucus-secreting goblet cells.

In chronic inflammatory conditions the ciliated epithelium becomes replaced by stratified cells, which are non-ciliated. This metaplasia may also occur following prolonged intubation of the trachea and tracheostomy.

Multiple-choice questions: Anatomy

1. The birth canal is innervated by the:
    a) pudendal nerve
    b) femoral nerve
    c) obturator nerve
    d) ilioinguinal nerve
    e) genitofemoral nerve.
2. Laryngeal motor innervation is from the following:
    a) glossopharyngeal nerve
    b) internal laryngeal nerve
    c) recurrent laryngeal nerve
    d) iliohypoglossal nerve
    e) superior laryngeal nerve.
3. In a 2-year-old child:
    a) the narrowest point of the trachea is the cricoid ring
    b) fluid requirements are 100 mL/kg per day
    c) blood volume is 50 mL/kg
    d) chest wall compliance is decreased compared to the adult
    e) there is increased platelet function.
4. The right lung has:
    a) one fissure
    b) no Sibson's fascia
    c) a direct relationship to the azygos vein
    d) two pulmonary veins
    e) seven bronchopulmonary segments.
5. The following are intimately related to the neck of a femoral hernia:
    a) pubic tubercle
    b) inguinal ligament
    c) inferior epigastric artery
    d) femoral vein
    e) femoral artery.
6. The coeliac plexus is related:
    a) anteriorly to the crura of the diaphragm
    b) anteriorly to the inferior vena cava
    c) anteriorly to the aorta
    d) to the L3 vertebra
    e) posteriorly to the pancreas.
7. For amputation at mid-thigh the following nerves must be blocked:
    a) obturator
    b) femoral

    c) sciatic

    d) genitofemoral

    e) lateral cutaneous nerve of the thigh.

8. The recurrent laryngeal nerve supplies:

    a) sensation below the cords

    b) the intrinsic muscles of the pharynx

    c) the cricothyroid muscle

    d) the inferior constrictor

    e) the epiglottis.

9. The following cross the 1st rib:

    a) the vagus nerve

    b) the subclavian artery

    c) the supratentorial membrane

    d) the T1 nerve root

    e) the sympathetic chain.

10. Concerning the cervical sympathetic chain:

    a) it terminates as a plexus around the internal carotid artery

    b) the cervical cord gives grey rami to the cervical chain which relays and distributes with the cervical nerves

    c) the middle cervical ganglion is a constant feature

    d) the inferior cervical and the first thoracic ganglia may fuse

    e) it is the site of relay for post-ganglionic fibres to the upper limb.

11. Concerning the femoral nerve:

    a) it arises from the L2, L3 and L4 spinal segments

    b) it lies lateral to the femoral artery at the inguinal ligament

    c) it supplies the lateral aspect of the thigh

    d) total block allows arthroscopy of the knee to be performed

    e) block relieves pain from a fractured femur.

12. The right main bronchus:

    a) has the pulmonary artery as a superior relation

    b) is 5 cm long

    c) is superior to the azygos vein

    d) gives off the middle lobar bronchus which divides into superior and inferior branches

    e) bifurcates with upper and lower branches.

13. The trachea:

    a) is 1.5–2 cm in diameter

    b) begins at C4 and ends at T6

    c) is supplied entirely by the bronchial arteries

    d) is lined by transitional epithelium

    e) is narrowest at the level of the cricoid in a child.

14. The parietal pleura at the lung apex:
    a) is attached to the medial one-third of clavicle
    b) rises 2.5 cm above the neck of the 1st rib
    c) is grooved by the subclavian vein
    d) is closely related to the phrenic nerve
    e) is attached to the transverse process of C7.

Answers to multiple-choice questions

1.	a) True;	b) False;	c) False;	d) True;	e) True
2.	a) False;	b) False;	c) True;	d) False;	e) True
3.	a) True;	b) True;	c) False;	d) False;	e) False
4.	a) False;	b) False;	c) True;	d) True;	e) False
5.	a) True;	b) True;	c) False;	d) True;	e) False
6.	a) True;	b) False;	c) True;	d) False;	e) True
7.	a) True;	b) True;	c) True;	d) False;	e) True
8.	a) True;	b) False;	c) False;	d) False;	e) False
9.	a) False;	b) True;	c) False;	d) True;	e) False
10.	a) True;	b) True;	c) False;	d) True;	e) True
11.	a) True;	b) True;	c) False;	d) False;	e) True
12.	a) False;	b) False;	c) False;	d) False;	e) True
13.	a) True;	b) False;	c) False;	d) False;	e) True
14.	a) True;	b) False;	c) True;	d) True;	e) False

SECTION THREE

CARDIOTHORACIC ANAESTHESIA

1 Coronary artery bypass surgery

> Outline the anaesthetic management of a patient undergoing coronary artery bypass surgery.

Coronary artery bypass graft (CABG) surgery is one of the most common operations performed in the world. With the continued development of percutaneous transluminal revascularisation techniques, the population of patients presenting for open coronary surgery have more extensive disease, frequently with impaired left ventricular function and comorbid pathology.

Preoperative preparation

When assessing the patient preoperatively, special consideration should be given to elucidating the following:

*   *The severity of the coronary artery disease.* If the patient has a significant left main stem lesion then most of the left ventricle is in jeopardy if coronary perfusion falls.
*   *Ventricular function.* If ejection fraction is not measured there may be a subjective opinion in the cardiac catheter report (not always reliable). A history of multiple infarcts is likely to result in impaired ventricular function.
*   The presence of comorbid disease:
    *   cerebrovascular disease
    *   respiratory disease
    *   renal dysfunction
    *   diabetes mellitus
    *   peripheral vascular disease
    *   coagulopathy (may be drug-induced).

An explanation should be given of anticipated events, including postoperative assisted ventilation.

An anxiolytic, amnesic premedicant should be prescribed and is frequently combined with an H_2 antagonist or an ATPase inhibitor. Aspirin and clopidogrel should be discontinued 7–10 days preoperatively. All cardiac medications should be continued up to, and including, the morning of the operation, with the exception of angiotensin converting enzyme (ACE) inhibitors and digoxin. Added oxygen should be administered for the transfer to the anaesthetic room.

Monitoring

The following are routine for all CABG operations:
*   5-lead ECG
*   invasive blood pressure monitoring

- pulse oximetry
- capnography
- central venous access and pressure monitoring
- core temperature (nasopharyngeal).

A large-bore venous cannula should be inserted prior to induction of anaesthesia. There is no compelling evidence to support the routine use of a pulmonary artery catheter, and the latter is rarely necessary for routine CABG surgery in the absence of severe ventricular dysfunction. Transoesophageal echocardiography (TOE, TEE) is being used increasingly and provides useful information regarding the structural integrity of the heart, ventricular function, volume status and the occurrence of regional wall motion abnormalities (RWMA) which may represent ischaemia.

Induction and maintenance of anaesthesia

A balanced anaesthetic technique is usually employed. A combination of etomidate, fentanyl (10–15 µg/kg) and muscle relaxant (pancuronium or rocuronium) provides a stable haemodynamic induction. Maintenance of anaesthesia can be achieved with an inhalational agent (usually isoflurane) or a propofol infusion.

Events that cause maximum stimulation include laryngoscopy, skin incision, sternotomy and sternal spread. Stages of lower level intensity occur pre-incision, and during internal mammary artery and saphenous vein dissection, cardiopulmonary bypass (CPB) and post-CPB. Anaesthetic depth is adjusted accordingly.

Pre-CPB

Prior to initiating cardiopulmonary bypass, heparin (initial dose 300 IU/kg) is administered to ensure total anticoagulation. An activated clotting time (ACT) (normal range 105–160 s) of greater than 480 seconds should be achieved prior to CPB.

After heparinisation, the surgeon cannulates the ascending aorta, proximal to the innominate artery and distal to the proposed site for the vein grafts. The venous cannula is usually a single two-stage cannula (right atrial basket and IVC tip) and it is inserted via the right atrial appendage.

Cardiopulmonary bypass

Blood bypasses the heart and lungs and drains by gravity, via the venous cannula, from the central veins into a reservoir on the bypass machine. It then passes through the oxygenator and filters, to remove debris, before being actively pumped at arterial pressure into the ascending aorta. Positive-pressure ventilation is discontinued for the duration of total CPB.

CABG surgery with CPB can be performed with or without cardioplegia:

(i) Cardioplegia and mild to moderate hypothermia

Total CPB is initiated with the empty heart still beating. Ventricular fibrillation (VF) may be induced spontaneously by hypothermia. The ascending aorta is cross-clamped and cardioplegia (solution with a high potassium concentration that arrests the heart in diastole) is infused proximal to the clamp into the aortic root and hence anterograde down the coronary arteries. Cardioplegia may be crystalloid or blood and can be administered warm or cold. The distal ends of the saphenous vein grafts are constructed on the diseased coronary arteries, followed by the internal mammary artery anastomosis to the left anterior descending (LAD) artery. As the final distal anastomosis is being constructed the patient is rewarmed. The aorta is then unclamped and a partial aortic side-clamp is applied to the side wall of the ascending aorta to allow attachment of the proximal ends of the vein grafts whilst cardioplegia is washed out of the coronary circulation. As the heart rewarms, VF or spontaneous contractions return. When sufficiently warm the heart is defibrillated.

(ii) Fibrillation/defibrillation without hypothermia

The heart is not actively cooled but the temperature is allowed to drift down passively. The aorta is cross-clamped and ventricular fibrillation is induced electrically. A distal anastomosis is constructed on the fibrillating heart and then the aorta is unclamped. If the heart does not defibrillate spontaneously with the resumption of coronary blood flow, a direct DC shock is administered and the proximal end is constructed as detailed in (i) above. This sequence of events is repeated for each graft.

Monitoring during CPB

The ACT should be maintained >480s with 5000- to 10000-unit increments of heparin. Blood gas, acid/base and electrolyte levels must be monitored regularly throughout the bypass period. Urine output is reduced during hypothermia; polyuria is often seen on rewarming due to haemodilution and mannitol in the bypass circuit.

Maintenance of anaesthesia during CPB

This can be achieved by a propofol infusion, benzodiazepines or an inhalational agent (attach vaporiser to oxygenator gas inlet).

Adjusting systemic pressure during CPB

- Vary the pump flow rate. This should not be used as the primary method as increased flow rates to compensate for a low systemic vascular resistance (SVR) cause unnecessary blood trauma.
- Increase the SVR. This is the main method for treating hypotension, using an α_1 agonist such as metaraminol or phenylephrine.

- Decrease the SVR:
  - α-adrenergic antagonists (e.g.phentolamine)
  - direct vasodilators (e.g. glyceryl trinitrate or sodium nitroprusside)
  - volatile anaesthetics administered via the oxygenator gas inlet line
  - narcotics.

Fluid management during CPB

The fluid that primes the bypass circuit is usually entirely crystalloid. If the patient has a very low body surface area or there is pre-CPB anaemia, blood can be added to the prime to avoid excessive haemodilution. Haemodilution reduces during CPB owing to free water and electrolytes being filtered by the kidneys and redistribution of fluid by diffusion into interstitial tissue spaces as oedema. This results in a progressive elevation of haemoglobin (Hb) during CPB. Excessive circulating blood volume can be reduced by:

- inducing a diuresis with frusemide
- ultrafiltration (UF) – a UF device is added to the bypass circuit.

Weaning from CPB

Before discontinuing CPB it is essential to check the following:

1. *Temperature.* Core temperature should be greater than 37°C to avoid hypo-thermia after active rewarming is discontinued, due to equilibration of cooler, less well perfused areas with the warmer, better perfused tissues.
2. *Heart rate.* A rate of 70–90 bpm is usually required; abnormal left ventric-ular stiffness prevents the normal increase in stroke volume at lower heart rates. Epicardial pacing is employed to treat asystole or bradycardia. DC cardioversion should be used to restore sinus rhythm in the presence of fast atrial tachyarrhythmias.
3. *Ventilation.* The lungs must be fully reinflated and intermittent positive-pressure ventilation (IPPV) commenced. Nitrous oxide must be avoided after CPB (avoid expansion of intravascular bubbles).
4. *Haemoglobin.* Should be greater than 7 g/dL.
5. *Arterial blood gases.* Extreme acidosis and potassium levels must be cor-rected.

   Protamine should be drawn up, and appropriate inotrope or antihypertens-ive/anti-ischaemic infusions should be available as required.

Predictors of difficult weaning from CPB

The following are predictors:

- preoperative ejection fraction less than 35%
- prolonged CPB (over 3 hours)
- incomplete revascularisation
- incomplete myocardial preservation during CPB
- ongoing or evolving myocardial ischaemia in the pre-CPB period.

Sequence of events during weaning from CPB

1. *Retard venous return to the pump.* As the heart fills it begins to eject.
2. *Lower pump flow into the aorta.*
3. *Terminate bypass.* Once the heart is generating an adequate systolic pressure (90–100 mmHg) at an acceptable preload with a pump flow rate of 1 L/min or less, the pump is stopped and both cannulae are clamped.

Increments of 100 mL of pump blood from the venous reservoir are infused via the aortic cannula to increase preload and optimise cardiac output. If blood pressure and cardiac output do not alter with volume infusion, then the heart is probably at the top of the Frank–Starling curve and further blood boluses are unlikely to be of benefit and may overfill the heart. If blood pressure does rise this is likely to be due to an increase in cardiac output and more volume is likely to be beneficial.

2 Problems in 24-hour period after CABG

List the potential postoperative problems in the first 24 hours after coronary artery bypass grafting.

Cardiovascular complications

1. Hypotension due to low cardiac output:
   myocardial ischaemia
   perioperative myocardial infarction
   inadequate preload
   increased afterload
   arrhythmias
   tamponade
   fluid overload.
2. Hypotension due to low systemic vascular resistance (SVR):
   vasodilatation with rewarming
   drug or transfusion reactions
   excessive vasodilator usage
   anaemia
   hyperthermia
   sepsis.
3. Hypertension
   pain and/or anxiety
   residual neuromuscular blockade
   iatrogenic hypertension
   pre-existing hypertension
   fluid overload
   shivering.
4. Arrhythmias
   electrolyte abnormalities (potassium, magnesium, calcium)
   myocardial ischaemia
   myocardial hypertrophy
   hypothermia
   acid/base abnormalities
   hypoxia
   hypertarbia
   tamponade.
5. Conduction abnormalities.
6. Pulmonary hypertension.

Respiratory complications

1. Postoperatively there is:
   reduced total lung capacity, inspiratory capacity and functional residual
      capacity (FRC)
   reduced total lung compliance (75% of baseline)
   left lower lobe atelectasis in at least 50% of patients
   increased intrapulmonary shunting
   increased extravascular lung water
   increased work of breathing.
2. Failure to wean from ventilatory support, hypoxia and/or hypercapnia may
   occur secondary to:
   atelectasis
   increased secretions
   pneumothorax
   hydrothorax
   bronchospasm
   oversedation
   incomplete reversal of neuromuscular block
   pre-existing respiratory disease.

Central nervous system complications

1. Type I neurological injury (major focal neurological deficits, stupor or
   coma).
2. Type II neurological injury (deterioration in intellectual function).
3. Inadequate pain relief.

Metabolic complications

1. Diabetes mellitus.
2. Acid/base abnormalities.

Renal complications

Renal failure.

Surgical complications

1. Haemorrhage.
2. Tamponade.
3. Acute graft occlusion.

Miscellaneous complications

1. Shivering.
2. Hypothermia.

3 Management in 24-hour period after CABG

> Outline the management of a patient during the first 24 hours following coronary artery bypass grafting.

Transfer of the patient from the operating theatre to the intensive care unit is a critical stage and may be complicated by cardiorespiratory decompensation. Full monitoring must be ensured. Comprehensive handover of pertinent pre-operative and intraoperative information must be given to the receiving staff.

Respiratory system

Check:
- the breathing circuit
- the adequacy of positive-pressure ventilation (auscultation, pulse oximetry, capnography, arterial blood gases)
- initial ventilator settings:
  - F_IO_2 of 0.5
  - PEEP of 5 mmHg
  - tidal volume of 10–12 mL/kg
  - respiratory rate of 10–12 breaths per minute
  - I:E ratio of 1:2.

A chest x-ray can be requested to look for correct endotracheal tube placement, position of central line, cardiac and mediastinal widening, pulmonary oedema, pleural effusion, pneumo- and haemothoraces and atelectasis.

Weaning from the ventilator should commence within 2 hours of the end of surgery provided the following criteria are satisfied:
- haemodynamic stability
- haemostasis
- normothermia
- no neurological dysfunction
- satisfactory arterial blood gases
- normal ventilatory parameters.

Treatment of postoperative respiratory complications is directed towards the cause (see list of postoperative respiratory complications above). Postextubation atelectasis is usually managed satisfactorily with either continuous or biphasic positive airway pressure (CPAP, BiPAP).

Cardiovascular system
Check:
* heart rate
* rhythm (lead II)
* evidence of ischaemia (lead V_5; compare with preoperative ECG)
* systemic blood pressure
* central venous ± pulmonary artery pressure and pulmonary capillary wedge pressure (PCWP)
* peripheral pulses and temperature
* urine output
* acid/base status
* pacemaker functioning, if present.

A postoperative 12-lead ECG should be performed to look for ischaemia, conduction abnormalities and arrhythmias.

Management of complications
1. *Low cardiac output* (cardiac index $<2.5 \, L/min/m^2$)

   Perioperative myocardial infarction occurs in up to 10% of cases. Postoperative myocardial ischaemia occurs with incomplete revascularisation or graft occlusion. It may require inotropic support (a) *pharmacologically* with a β_1 agonist (e.g. dopamine, adrenaline) or a phosphodiesterase inhibitor (e.g. milrinone); or (b) *mechanically* (intra-aortic balloon pump, left ventricular assist device).

2. *Reduced preload*

   This occurs with inadequate fluid and blood replacement and may be due to continuing blood loss. Any existing coagulopathy must be corrected. If bleeding persists the patient may need to undergo an exploratory reopening of the chest.

3. *Increased afterload, due to a raised SVR, in combination with poor ventricular function*

   This may lead to pump failure. Afterload reduction with vasodilator therapy (GTN, SNP) may improve cardiac output.

4. *Arrhythmias*

   Bradycardia can be corrected by temporary pacing with epicardial pacing wires sited intraoperatively. Supraventricular tachyarrhythmias resulting in haemodynamic deterioration should be corrected with a DC cardioversion.

5. *Mechanical causes*

   Mechanical causes of pump failure include cardiac tamponade and tension pneumothorax which require urgent chest opening and insertion of an appropriately sited intercostal drain respectively.

Hypotension due to a low SVR frequently responds to expansion of the circulating volume. However, it may be necessary to commence a noradrenaline infusion.

Hypertension may be due to pain, shivering, incomplete reversal of muscle relaxation or anxiety. If these causes have been excluded, administration of a vasodilator (e.g. GTN, SNP) and/or a beta-blocker may be necessary.

Treatment of postoperative arrhythmias is directed at the cause (see above). Atrial fibrillation (AF) occurs in up to 30% of patients, usually on the second or third postoperative day. Restarting beta-blockers in the postoperative period reduces the incidence of postoperative AF. If DC cardioversion is not possible or is unsuccessful, an intravenous infusion of amiodarone can be commenced to control the ventricular rate.

Central nervous system

Sedation is usually provided by intravenous propofol. Alternatively, boluses or an infusion of midazolam may be used. Adequate postoperative analgesia reduces the incidence and severity of myocardial ischaemia. Intravenous boluses of morphine prior to commencement of patient-controlled analgesia (PCA) are frequently employed. Epidural analgesia is being used increasingly and provides excellent postoperative analgesia as well as reducing myocardial ischaemia by cardiac sympatholysis. Shivering is managed by effective rewarming and prevention of further temperature loss. Small boluses of intravenous pethidine and increased sedation may also be effective.

Metabolism

Postoperative hyperglycaemia occurs frequently in diabetic and non-diabetic patients and requires intravenous insulin infusion.

Acid/base abnormalities are common. Alteration in ventilatory parameters may be necessary for respiratory acidosis/alkalosis. Optimisation of cardiac and renal function helps to prevent metabolic acidosis. The latter may be due to splanchnic hypoperfusion during CPB and may persist for 24–48 hours.

Kidney function

Postoperative renal dysfunction (creatinine $>175\,\mu$mol/L or increase above baseline of more than $60\,\mu$mol/l) occurs in up to 8% of patients. Of these, 18% require renal support. If the preoperative creatinine is above $220\,\mu$mol/L, 40–50% require renal replacement therapy. The overall mortality among patients developing renal dysfunction is 19%. Haemofiltration may be required to control volume overload or electrolyte abnormalities.

Surgical complications

Profound haemorrhage may occur from a suture line or a cannulation site and necessitate return to theatre for exploratory sternotomy. Any coagulation abnormalities, detected by activated clotting time (ACT), thromboelastography (TEG), platelet count or formal clotting studies, must be corrected urgently. It may be necessary to perform the sternotomy in the ICU if bleeding is profound and the patient is unstable.

Cardiac tamponade can occur with excessive mediastinal bleeding. Raised right atrial pressure, tachycardia, arrhythmias, equalisation of left and right atrial pressures, low cardiac output, increasing metabolic acidosis and a fall in urinary output may be seen. Widening of the cardiac shadow on chest x-ray and compression of the heart seen on echocardiography allied to a high index of suspicion confirm the diagnosis. Immediate surgical intervention is essential.

4 Oesophagectomy

> Outline the anaesthetic management of a patient undergoing an oesophagectomy for carcinoma of the oesophagus.

The incidence of carcinoma of the oesophagus is increasing. The overall prognosis is poor as presentation is usually late in the course of the disease. Five-year survival in patients undergoing oesophagectomy is around 25%. Preoperative chemotherapy for surgical candidates is currently being assessed.

Patients usually present in the seventh decade and the tumour is more common in males. The lower oesophagus is affected in 50%, the middle-third in 35% and the upper-third in 15%. Lymphatic involvement is present in 60% of operative cases. Direct invasion of local vital structures can result in recurrent laryngeal and phrenic nerve palsies, tracheo-oesophageal fistula, empyema, lung abscess, pneumonia, pericarditis and superior vena caval obstruction.

Preoperative assessment and preparation

Preoperative anaemia, dehydration and electrolyte abnormalities should be corrected. Parenteral nutrition may be necessary in the severely cachectic patient. An acute chest infection secondary to aspiration of oesophageal contents will require preoperative antibiotics and physiotherapy. If there is evidence of chronic pulmonary damage, formal lung function testing must be performed. As the patient is likely to be elderly, unrelated cardiovascular disease, renal impairment, cerebrovascular disease and diabetes mellitus should be excluded. Therefore all patients due to undergo an oesophagectomy should have the following performed:
- full blood count
- urea, creatinine and electrolytes tests
- liver function tests and clotting profile
- blood glucose test
- group and cross matching
- chest radiography
- chest CT scan
- ECG.

Surgical techniques

There are three main types of surgical procedure.

Middle- and lower-third oesophageal tumours

The Ivor Lewis procedure is used. The first stage involves mobilisation of the stomach, with preservation of the right gastroepiploic artery, a pyloroplasty and widening of the oesophageal hiatus via an abdominal incision. The second stage consists of resection of the oesophageal tumour and anastomosis of the oesophageal remnant to the stomach, via a right posterolateral thoracotomy through the fourth or fifth intercostal space.

Tumours extending into the stomach

Oesophagogastrectomy can be performed for tumours extending into the stomach, via a left thoracoabdominal incision. The entire stomach and lower oesophagus are resected with the proximal jejunum anastomosed to the oesophageal remnant and a Roux-en-Y constructed.

High tumours

High tumours involve anastomosis between the oesophageal remnant and either colon or stomach in the neck. The stomach or colon is mobilised via an abdominal incision, and a right thoracotomy may be required for the oesophageal resection. This procedure is sometimes combined with a laryngectomy.

Anaesthetic technique

Premedication

As the patient frequently has dysphagia, oral medication may be unreliable and is frequently omitted. Neutralisation of gastric pH is not specifically indicated.

Induction of anaesthesia and airway management

During the investigative stage an endoscopy will have been performed and oesophageal obstruction can be assessed at this stage. If there is no history of dysphagia and no significant physical obstruction, then a rapid-sequence induction (RSI) is unnecessary. In all other circumstances, and if there is any doubt, then an RSI must be performed.

A left-sided double-lumen tube to allow collapse of the appropriate lung (right lung for Ivor Lewis and three-stage procedures, left lung for thoracoabdominal approach) should be used to facilitate surgical exposure of the tumour and creation of the anastomosis. A nasogastric tube must also be inserted.

Maintenance of anaesthesia

Factors influencing the choice of technique include the mode of analgesia employed and whether postoperative mechanical ventilation is planned. Use of an inhalation agent in an air/oxygen mixture, or total intravenous anaesthesia with propofol, in combination with muscle relaxation and thoracic epidural anaesthesia, provide satisfactory operating conditions and allow extubation of the patient's trachea at the end of the procedure. If it is not possible to employ a regional anaesthetic technique, then high-dose intravenous opioid must be used, with the increased likelihood of postoperative assisted ventilation.

Monitoring

Peroperative monitoring of the ECG, oxygen saturation, end-tidal carbon dioxide (ET_{CO_2}), blood pressure, central venous pressure, urine output, core temperature and ventilator parameters is mandatory. Blood pressure should be measured directly via an intra-arterial catheter. Periodic arterial blood gases should be measured during one-lung anaesthesia.

General measures

The pressure areas of a thin, cachectic patient are at particular risk and must be padded and protected. Heat losses during these long operations are considerable, so use of a warming blanket, heated intravenous fluids and humidification of inspired gases should be routine. Crystalloid fluid requirements are considerable and blood loss must be corrected promptly as hypovolaemia is poorly tolerated.

Intraoperative complications

Intraoperative complications include tracheal damage, pleural damage, and hypotension (hypovolaemia, regional anaesthetic block, and manipulation of the heart and great vessels). One-lung anaesthesia may result in hypoxaemia, and high inspired oxygen levels may be required (this does not alter the depth of anaesthesia if nitrous oxide is avoided). Cardiac output must be optimised and correct positioning of the double-lumen tube assured. On closure of the chest the collapsed lung must be reinflated completely.

Postoperative management

Postoperative care should be conducted in a high-dependency unit or an ICU in the infrequent situation where postoperative assisted ventilation is required. Measures outlined above must be continued in the postoperative phase to correct hypothermia and hypovolaemia. Fluid requirements are high and fluid replacement is guided by invasive pressure and temperature monitoring, urinary output and urinary and blood laboratory investigations. Parenteral feeding is initiated postoperatively. Provided there is no leak demonstrated on barium swallow, eating can be recommenced after five days.

Pulmonary complications are very common, and are due to the acute effects of thoracotomy on respiratory function, and pulmonary damage from chronic aspiration preoperatively. Optimal analgesia, physiotherapy and prompt treatment of infection with intravenous antibiotics will help to limit complications. A mini-tracheostomy may be required to clear tracheal secretions, and continuous positive airway pressure (CPAP) reduces the incidence of basal atelectasis. Non-invasive ventilation can sometimes be employed to obviate the need for reintubation.

Anastomotic breakdown results in mediastinitis and is associated with high morbidity and mortality. It occurs most commonly between the fourth and seventh postoperative days, presenting as chest pain, pyrexia, bile-stained drainage from the mediastinal drain, arrhythmias or respiratory failure.

5 Physiology of one-lung ventilation (OLV)

Outline the physiology of one-lung ventilation.

One-lung ventilation is employed to:
*   enable unilateral ventilation if the contralateral airways are to be opened
*   prevent secretions, pus or blood spilling from one side to the other
*   facilitate surgery.

Distribution of pulmonary blood flow

The pulmonary circulation is a low-pressure low-resistance system. Distribution of pulmonary blood flow is determined by the effects of gravity and by the resistance of the blood vessels. Approximately 40% of total pulmonary vascular resistance (PVR) is due to the resistance of intra-alveolar vessels (capillaries) which is determined by:
*   pulmonary artery pressure
*   pulmonary venous pressure
*   intra-alveolar pressure.

The remaining 60% of the PVR is from the extra-alveolar vessels (hilar vessels and the smaller vessels situated within the lung parenchyma). The resistance of the extra-alveolar vessels is determined by the difference between the intravascular pressure and the pressure in the surrounding interstitial space. The latter is determined by regional lung volume, the elastic recoil of the surrounding lung tissue and local pleural pressure. They are also affected by changes in autonomic tone.

Distribution of ventilation

Transpulmonary pressure (the difference between alveolar and pleural pressure) is responsible for lung expansion. The distribution of ventilation in a normal lung during a spontaneous breath is governed mainly by the pressure/volume (P–V) relationship (compliance) of the lungs.

The alveoli in the non-dependent parts of the lung have a higher resting volume than those in the dependent zones. However, for a given increase in transpulmonary pressure there is a greater expansion in the dependent alveoli than in the non-dependent alveoli because the former are on a steeper part of the pressure/volume curve.

General anaesthesia

Under general anaesthesia, both lungs lose volume and there is a reduction in functional residual capacity (FRC). In the lateral decubitus position this alters the position of both lungs on the P–V curve. In contrast to the awake situation, the non-dependent lung is situated on the steeper part of the curve and there-fore receives more ventilation per unit change in pressure. The pulmonary blood flow is greater to the lower, dependent lung owing to the effect of gravity, so contributing to ventilation–perfusion (V–Q) mismatch. Muscle relaxation and paralysis of the diaphragm in the lateral decubitus position results in the lateral pressure of the abdominal contents being transmitted directly to the pleural space which, in addition to compression by the heart and mediastinal structures, causes dependent zone atelectasis and a further decrease in dependent zone ventilation. Ventilation to the upper lung is increased further with opening of the hemithorax and removal of the constraints imposed by the chest wall.

With the institution of one-lung ventilation, the (preferential) ventilation to the upper lung ceases. Pulmonary blood flow continues to the non-ventil-ated upper lung, resulting in a 'true' shunt (V/Q = 0). Within a few minutes the pulmonary blood to the collapsed lung no longer takes up oxygen, the rate being determined by the volume of oxygen in the alveoli and the magnitude of the blood flow. This relatively poorly oxygenated mixed venous blood mixes with oxygenated blood from the lower lung in the left atrium, causing venous admixture and a lowering of the arterial oxygen tension. This effect is greater if the right lung is collapsed. Other causes of venous admixture include:

- areas in the dependent lung that are less well ventilated, so creating further V–Q mismatch
- a fall in cardiac output resulting in a decreased mixed venous oxygen sat-uration (haemorrhage, arrhythmias, high inflation pressure, PEEP to depen-dent lung, manipulation of mediastinal structures impeding venous return).

The *shunt equation* indicates what proportion of total pulmonary blood flow would have bypassed ventilated alveoli to produce the given arterial blood gas values:

$$Q_s/Q_t = (C_cO_2 - C_aO_2)/(C_cO_2 - C_{\bar{v}}O_2)$$

where Q_s = flow through shunt, Q_t = cardiac output, C_cO_2 = oxygen content in pulmonary end-capillary blood, C_aO_2 = oxygen content in arterial blood, and $C_{\bar{v}}O_2$ = oxygen content in mixed venous blood.

Venous admixture increases from approximately 20% during two-lung ven-tilation to 30–40% during OLV.

The changes in carbon dioxide clearance with OLV are relatively minor and of less importance than those of oxygenation. If both lungs are normal, the minute-volume required during two-lung ventilation results in similar $P\text{CO}_2$ levels when delivered to only one lung. However, the ventilated lung must be able to accept the increased tidal volume without an undue increase in infla-tion pressure, which would otherwise result in an increased alveolar dead-space. If the ventilated lung is diseased it may not be able to excrete the entire carbon dioxide load.

Hypoxic pulmonary vasoconstriction (HPV) minimises hypoxaemia by diverting blood away from poorly oxygenated alveoli to better ventilated areas of the lung. In the absence of hypoxia there is little vascular tone. However, if there is a reduction in alveolar Po_2 to 8 kPa, the smaller pulmonary arterioles ($<$500 μm) constrict and reduce flow to the hypoxic area of the lung. The reduction in blood flow is usually complete within 10 minutes. HPV is inhibited by:

- high or low pulmonary vascular pressures
- high left atrial pressure
- vasodilators
- hypocarbia
- handling of the lung
- possibly volatile anaesthetic agents (evidence in animal experiments but not convincingly demonstrated in humans).

HPV is not inhibited by intravenous anaesthetic agents but no overall benefit has been demonstrated in terms of arterial oxygenation or shunt reduction.

If the non-ventilated non-dependent lung is significantly diseased, the blood supply may already be significantly reduced by HPV and physical means (collapse, consolidation, tumour infiltration), and that lung may have been contributing little to overall gas exchange. In this circumstance, OLV will have little effect on oxygenation.

6 One-lung ventilation: indications

List the indications for one-lung ventilation (OLV).

- Bronchopleural fistula
- Pulmonary suppurative disease – abscess
- Bronchiectasis
- Endobronchial haemorrhage
- Lung transplantation
- Bronchial transection/tear
- Bronchoplastic surgery (e.g. sleeve resection)
- Bullous lung disease
- Lung cyst
- Undrained pneumothorax
- Pulmonary resection (lobectomy, pneumonectomy)
- Thoracoscopic surgery
- Oesophageal surgery
- Pleurectomy
- Surgery for thoracic aortic disease
- Spinal surgery.

7 One-lung ventilation: technique

Describe your technique for one-lung ventilation (OLV).

Equipment

The device options for achieving one-lung ventilation are
- double-lumen tube (plastic or resterilisable rubber)
- bronchial blocker
- single-lumen endobronchial tube
- Fogarty embolectomy catheter
- Univent tube (combined endotracheal tube and bronchial blocker).

The double-lumen tube (DLT) is by far the most common device used for one-lung ventilation. Bronchial blockers are used rarely nowadays and only in specialist centres. In adults with small airways or abnormal tracheobronchial anatomy, a single-lumen endobronchial tube may be used. In children, a Fogarty embolectomy catheter or a normal endotracheal tube can be guided into the relevant main bronchus with the aid of fibreoptic bronchoscopy.

The Univent tube consists of a single-lumen endotracheal tube with a moveable bronchial blocker in a narrow compartment of its anterior wall. This device has not gained universal acceptance and is appropriate only for specialist centres.

Left- or right-sided DLT?

The DLT should be placed in the main bronchus of the lung contralateral to the side of surgery for lung resection. This avoids the need to withdraw the tube prior to completion of pneumonectomy or upper lobectomy on that side. Although lobectomy may be the planned procedure, not infrequently it is necessary to convert this into a pneumonectomy in order to resect the tumour in its entirety. As the length of bronchus proximal to the upper lobe orifice is greater on the left side, a left-sided DLT is often selected for surgery not involving lung resection. However, protection of the ventilated lung from aspiration or spillage is more reliably achieved by intubation of the main bronchus of the ventilated lung. Whichever sided tube is chosen, correct positioning of the DLT should be confirmed by fibreoptic bronchoscopy.

Choice of tube size

Non-disposable rubber Robertshaw tubes (or their equivalent) are made in three sizes: small, medium and large. Disposable plastic tubes are measured in Charriere (Ch) gauge sizes (equivalent to French gauge) and are available in sizes 28 (left), 35, 37, 39 and 41.

The largest tube that can be passed easily through the vocal cords should be selected. This is usually a large Robertshaw tube or a size 39 or 41 disposable plastic tube for a male, or a medium-sized Robertshaw tube or a size 37 or 39 plastic disposable tube for a female. Larger tubes are easier to place successfully, present less resistance to gas flow, and allow easier suction of secretions.

Checking the position of the DLT

The optimal technique for checking the position of a DLT is with the aid of a fibreoptic bronchoscope. The latter is passed initially down the tracheal limb to check the position of the bronchial cuff, which should be seen just distal to the carina in the relevant main bronchus. The bronchoscope is then passed through the bronchial limb to ensure that the endobronchial extension is not obstructing the upper lobe bronchus. The left upper-lobe (LUL) bronchus should be visible distal to the tip of the endobronchial extension with a left-sided DLT; the right upper-lobe (RUL) orifice should be visible through the ventilation slot for the RUL with a right-sided DLT.

Correct tube placement can be checked clinically as follows:

1. Inflate the tracheal cuff, auscultate both lung fields and check end-tidal CO_2.
2. Clamp the limb of the connector connecting to the bronchial limb and gently inflate the bronchial cuff until no leak is audible from the bronchial lumen open to the atmosphere.
3. Auscultate both lung fields to check that there are breath sounds only on the bronchial side (including over the upper lobe).
4. Unclamp the bronchial limb and close it to the atmosphere. Clamp the limb of the connector connecting to the tracheal limb and open the tracheal lumen to the atmosphere. Check there is no audible leak from the tracheal lumen and auscultate for breath sounds over the ventilated lung. Peak airway pressure should not exceed 35 cmH$_2$O.

Initiation of one-lung ventilation

The overall aims are:

* maintenance of adequate arterial oxygen saturation
* collapse of the non-dependent non-ventilated lung
* ventilation of all areas of dependent lung with satisfactory mean and peak inspiratory pressures.

Although maintenance of normocapnia is ideal, and usually achieved, a degree of permissive hypercapnia for the duration of OLV may be necessary and is unlikely to be harmful.

Two-lung ventilation is continued until pleurotomy. On initiation of OLV, the F_IO_2 should be increased to 1.0. It is usually possible to maintain the same tidal volume and ventilation rate. Peak inspiratory pressure (PIP) inevitably increases. If it exceeds 35 cmH$_2$O, a reduced tidal volume and higher ventilatory rate should be employed.

High PIP is associated with alveolar damage and barotrauma whereas high mean inspiratory pressure (MIP) has a detrimental effect on cardiac output and may increase the shunt to the non-ventilated lung. Increasing the I:E ratio reduces PIP but will increase MIP. Typical initial settings are:

- tidal volume of 10 mL/kg
- ventilation rate of 12/min
- I:E of 1:2
- F_1O_2 of 1.0.

If there is not a significant fall in S_aO_2 after 10 minutes, the F_1O_2 should be reduced accordingly.

There is some evidence that pressure-controlled ventilation may be preferable to volume-controlled ventilation with lower mean intrapulmonary pressures and better preserved arterial oxygenation.

8 One-lung ventilation: problems

> **What problems are commonly encountered with one-lung ventilation (OLV)?**

Common problems with OLV are:
* hypoxaemia
* inadvertent ventilation of the non-dependent lung
* failure of the non-dependent lung to collapse.

Hypoxaemia
Mechanical problems
Check the anaesthetic machine, the breathing circuit and the position of the DLT. Correct any leaks and aspirate any blood or secretions obstructing the airway.

Inadequate cardiac output
Optimise the relevant haemodynamic parameters. Consider transoesophageal echocardiography (TOE, TEE) if you are unsure of the cause of a low cardiac output.

Shunt and/or V–Q mismatch in ventilated lung
1. Review ventilation settings.
2. Provide continuous positive airway pressure (CPAP) to the non-dependent non-ventilated lung (5 cmH$_2$O) to improve oxygenation of pulmonary blood perfusing the non-ventilated lung. Close liaison with the surgeon is important to avoid hindering surgery as much as possible.
3. Provide positive end-expiratory pressure (PEEP) to the ventilated lung. The beneficial effects of airway recruitment and increasing end-expiratory volume may be offset by the increase in mean intrapulmonary pressure and pulmonary vascular resistance shunting more blood to the non-ventilated lung. PEEP may also reduce cardiac output.
4. Insufflate oxygen into the non-ventilated lung.
5. Start intermittent re-expansion of the non-dependent lung after consultation with the surgeon. This will provide adequate oxygen saturation for up to 10 minutes after resumption of OLV.
6. Start high-frequency jet ventilation via an endotracheal portion of the DLT.
7. Clamp the pulmonary artery supplying the lung to be resected at the earliest opportunity.

If these measures fail to resolve the hypoxaemia, resumption of two-lung ventilation and manual retraction of the upper lung will have to be employed.

Inadvertent ventilation of the non-dependent lung

Check that:
- the correct limb to the DLT has been clamped
- the bronchial cuff is adequately inflated and has not ruptured
- the DLT is correctly positioned with a fibreoptic bronchoscope (the endo-bronchial limb may be in the wrong main bronchus or may have become displaced proximal to the carina).

Failure of the non-dependent lung to collapse

Consider these possible causes:
- In patients with severe emphysema, lung deflation may take up to 15 minutes to occur owing to airway compression by the hyperinflated lungs.
- A tumour, inflammatory lesion or foreign body obstructing a proximal bronchus may likewise prevent rapid deflation of the lung. Airway secretions or blood should be aspirated.
- Pleural adhesions may need to be divided before the lung is able to collapse.
- Proximal herniation of the bronchial cuff above the carina, producing obstruction of the contralateral main bronchus, is easily identifiable with a fibreoptic bronchoscope.

9 Post-thoracotomy pain

> Discuss the management of post-thoracotomy pain.

Pain from a thoracotomy incision is more intense than from other sites owing to continuous chest wall movement with ventilation. The area is extensively innervated and a thoracotomy involves resection or trauma to ribs, periosteum, muscles, intercostal nerves, pericardium, pleura, lungs and the diaphragm. High-quality analgesia is required to:

- allow the patient to take deep inspiratory breaths and clear pulmonary secretions
- limit the stress response
- allow early mobilisation.

Postoperative pain relief must be discussed in detail with the patient. The importance of chest physiotherapy should be explained by an appropriately trained physiotherapist. If an Acute Pain Team is to supervise postoperative pain relief, they should also meet the patient preoperatively.

A full thoracotomy incision extends over the T2–T10 dermatomes, and chest drain insertion may be at a lower dermatomal level. In addition, shoulder pain may accompany that from the thoracotomy incision owing to retraction of the shoulder in the thoracotomy position and to diaphragmatic irritation. Nerve groups involved in the conduction of painful stimuli include the intercostal nerves, phrenic nerve (diaphragmatic pleura), vagus nerve (lung and mediastinal pleura) and the cervical spinal nerves (shoulder). The chosen analgesic technique may reflect the nature of the recovery facilities and the availability of appropriate medical and nursing personnel.

Options for treatment

The options available for the treatment of post-thoracotomy pain are as follows:

- *Local anaesthetic blocks*
  - local infiltration
  - intercostal nerve blocks
  - interpleural block
  - paravertebral block
  - thoracic epidural block
  - subarachnoid block.
- *Opioid analgesia*
  - oral
  - subcutaneous
  - intramuscular

- intravenous – boluses, continuous infusion or patient-controlled analgesia (PCA).
- *Non-steroidal anti-inflammatory drugs* (NSAIDS).
- *Miscellaneous*
  - transcutaneous electrical nerve stimulation (TENS)
  - cryoanalgesia
  - acupuncture
  - hypnotherapy.

Advantages and disadvantages

Although it is theoretically possible to perform a thoracotomy with local anaesthesia, this is not used for postoperative pain relief – other than for phrenic nerve blockade – owing to its short duration of action.

Intercostal nerve blocks
For
Easy to perform.

Against
- Relatively short duration of action. Although it is possible to insert a catheter for repeated injections or an infusion, the multiple levels required preclude this technique.
- Risk of systemic toxicity owing to the large volumes of local anaesthetic required over multiple levels.
- Risk of pneumothorax.
- Risk of intravascular injection.

Interpleural block
A catheter is inserted between the visceral and parietal pleurae. The mechanism of action is by widespread intercostal neural blockade. It is not commonly used as the sole analgesic technique.

For
Solitary injection site (cf. intercostal nerve blocks).

Against
- Distribution of local anaesthetic is posture-dependent. The patient must lie supine.
- 30–40% of the local anaesthetic is lost via the intercostal drains.
- Risk of pneumothorax.
- Risk of lung laceration or bronchopleural fistula with the 'blind' insertion technique.
- Analgesia is unpredictable.

Paravertebral block

This block can be administered by 'blind' percutaneous injection, or a catheter can be inserted in the paravertebral gutter by the surgeon under direct vision. This technique can provide satisfactory post-thoracotomy analgesia and may be gaining in popularity. However, it is less reliable than thoracic epidural analgesia.

For
- Blocks multiple intercostal nerves with a solitary injection.
- Less chance of spinal cord trauma than with an epidural.
- Less sympathetic block and less hypotension.

Against
- Requires large doses of local anaesthetic.
- Risk of pneumothorax.
- Risk of vascular injury.
- Risk of dural puncture.

Thoracic epidural analgesia

This technique is generally considered the gold standard for post-thoracotomy analgesia. Although the thoracic level should be used if administering epidural local anaesthetics, the lumbar route provides comparable levels of analgesia if solely using opiates.

For
- Provides excellent analgesia.
- Insertion of an epidural catheter allows an infusion to be continued for several days post-op.
- It is titratable.
- Improved coronary blood flow.
- Reduced stress response.

Against
- Can be technically difficult.
- Requires a high level of supervision by appropriately trained medical and nursing personnel.
- Risk of respiratory depression with opioids.
- Urinary retention (requires insertion of a urinary catheter).
- Opioids tend to produce pruritus.
- Risk of nerve/spinal cord damage with insertion.
- Risk of vascular damage and epidural haematoma.
- Risk of epidural abscess.
- Risk of dural puncture and associated headache.
- Can produce hypotension.

Subarachnoid block
This route is used much less commonly compared with the paravertebral and epidural routes.

For
- Rapid onset of action.
- Usually technically easy to perform.
- Less chance of causing neurological damage on insertion.

Against
The disadvantages include those listed above under thoracic epidural block, except for the risk of dural puncture. Also, the relatively short duration of action precludes its use in the setting of major thoracic surgery. Siting an intrathecal catheter for a continuous infusion is rarely, if ever, used nowadays.

Parenteral opioids
Although they are less effective at providing post-thoracotomy analgesia than regional anaesthetic techniques, parenteral opioids may be used in isolation. Side-effects include pruritus, urinary retention, nausea and vomiting, respiratory depression, drowsiness, dysphoria, bradycardia and hypotension.

Intramuscular opioids, once the mainstay of postoperative analgesia, provide inadequate pain relief unless used in a dose that is likely to cause unpleasant and dangerous side-effects.

Subcutaneous opioids can provide satisfactory analgesia but are subject to variable absorption in the postoperative setting. They are not commonly used.

Intravenous opioids can be used alone or in combination with a local anaesthetic block. They may be administered in a variety of ways:
- *Boluses*. Intermittent IV boluses provide barely better analgesia than IM opioids, with the inevitable peaks and troughs of serum concentrations resulting in variable analgesia.
- *Continuous infusion*. This provides better analgesia than boluses, with less fluctuation in serum concentration. Progressive sedation is a disadvantage.
- *Patient-controlled analgesia*. This is the optimum technique for administering opioids intravenously.

For
- There is good patient compliance and acceptability.
- There is flexibility.
- Relatively constant serum concentrations can be achieved with an acceptable incidence of side-effects.
- A lockout period reduces the risk of overdose.

Against
The main disadvantages of PCA opioids relate to the side-effects listed above.

Non-steroidal anti-inflammatory drugs (NSAIDS)
Drugs in this class have a major role to play in the setting of post-thoracotomy pain relief.

For
- They complement regional anaesthetic blocks.
- They are particularly useful for the relief of shoulder pain postoperatively which may not be within the range of the regional block.
- They reduce opioid consumption.

Against
- They tend to produce gastrointestinal erosions and ulceration.
- Platelet dysfunction may arise. However, this has not been demonstrated to increase postoperative bleeding significantly.
- There is a reduced renal blood flow and glomerular filtration rate.

Transcutaneous nerve stimulation
This is not a commonly employed postoperative analgesic technique. It is more useful for relief of chronic musculoskeletal pain.

For
- There are no serious side-effects.
- It may have an opioid-sparing effect.
- There is less nausea and vomiting.

Against
- It is contraindicated in the presence of a pacemaker.
- It cannot be used as the sole analgesic technique.

Cryoanalgesia
With the advent of more sophisticated techniques there is now little place for cryoanalgesia in managing post-thoracotomy pain. Rapid cooling of the inter-costal nerve by a cryoprobe placed as close as possible to the intercostal foramen results in long-term but ultimately reversible analgesia. Disadvantages that make this an inappropriate method of analgesia are:
- long-term neuralgia
- inadequacy as the sole means of analgesia
- possible permanent nerve damage.

In addition, long-term anaesthesia of thoracic dermatomes may be distressing.

Acupuncture
In the West this is rarely used for providing postoperative pain relief. In China the technique is used very effectively.

Multiple-choice questions: Cardiothoracic surgery

1. A peanut lodged in a child's main bronchus commonly shows:
   a) pneumonia
   b) lung collapse
   c) haemoptysis
   d) chronic cough
   e) emphysema.
2. Six hours after thoracotomy for oesophageal resection:
   a) vital capacity is reduced
   b) FRC is reduced
   c) peak expiratory flow is reduced
   d) venous admixture is reduced
   e) P_aO_2 on air is reduced.
3. Goldman Cardiac Risk criteria include:
   a) previous cardiac surgery
   b) mitral valve disease
   c) hypertension
   d) atrial fibrillation
   e) previous myocardial infarction.
4. During one-lung anaesthesia the P_aO_2 is influenced by:
   a) the amount of blood flow in the upper lung
   b) the cardiac output
   c) the mixed venous oxygen concentration
   d) the haematocrit
   e) the F_iO_2.
5. In one-lung ventilation, hypoxic vasoconstriction is enhanced by:
   a) volatile agents
   b) intravenous anaesthetics
   c) sodium nitroprusside
   d) administering oxygen to the non-dependent lung
   e) metabolic alkalosis.
6. In the normal pulmonary vascular bed:
   a) the mean pulmonary arterial pressure is half the mean aortic pressure
   b) the pulmonary vascular resistance is lower than the systemic vascular resistance
   c) there is always 50% of the blood volume
   d) the pulmonary capillary wedge pressure equals capillary pressure
   e) hypoxia causes dilatation of blood vessels.

7. Physiological right-to-left shunt (venous admixture) is:
   a) partly flow from bronchial veins into pulmonary veins
   b) partly from Thebesian veins
   c) 20% of total pulmonary blood flow
   d) mainly through giant subpleural capillaries
   e) increased during general anaesthesia.

8. Lung compliance is increased in:
   a) the presence of intra-alveolar fluid
   b) ARDS
   c) idiopathic pulmonary fibrosis
   d) emphysema
   e) fibrosing alveolitis.

9. Ventricular arrhythmias are more common in the presence of:
   a) hypokalaemia
   b) hypoxia
   c) thyrotoxicosis
   d) cardiopulmonary bypass and digoxin treatment
   e) essential hypertension.

10. During one-lung anaesthesia the following influence the arterial Po_2:
    a) haemoglobin concentration
    b) airway pressure
    c) the degree of perfusion of the non-ventilated lung
    d) inspired oxygen concentration
    e) blood pressure.

11. Pulmonary stenosis as an isolated finding is associated with:
    a) central cyanosis
    b) a large 'a' wave in the CVP waveform
    c) a loud P2
    d) a systolic murmur at the left sternal edge with a thrill
    e) a parasternal heave.

12. Rheumatoid arthritis is associated with:
    a) aortic valve disease
    b) pericardial effusion
    c) constrictive pericarditis
    d) renal failure
    e) tricuspid incompetence.

13. Fallot's tetralogy includes:
    a) pulmonary stenosis
    b) right ventricular hypertrophy
    c) overriding aorta
    d) atrial septal defect (ASD)
    e) patent ductus arteriosus (PDA).

14. Pulmonary arterial hypertension may be caused by:
   a) patent ductus arteriosus
   b) pulmonary regurgitation
   c) mitral stenosis
   d) recurrent pulmonary emboli
   e) hypoxaemia.
15. Radiographic enlargement of the pulmonary artery is seen in:
   a) atrial septal defect (ASD)
   b) ventricular septal defect (VSD)
   c) patent ductus arteriosus (PDA)
   d) Fallots' tetralogy
   e) pulmonary stenosis.
16. A large A–V shunt causes:
   a) increased cardiac output
   b) increased total systemic vascular resistance (SVR)
   c) cold extremities
   d) tachycardia
   e) heart failure.
17. Pulmonary hypertension is caused by:
   a) multiple pulmonary emboli
   b) mitral stenosis
   c) chronic obstructive airways disease
   d) volatile anaesthetic agents
   e) ascent to high altitude.
18. Coarctation of the aorta:
   a) is a congenital condition
   b) produces upper-limb hypertension
   c) may be associated with a displaced apex beat
   d) produces a diastolic murmur over the precordium
   e) produces skeletal abnormalities on a plain chest x-ray.
19. Atrial flutter:
   a) is caused most commonly by ischaemic heart disease
   b) is identified by 'f' waves at 20/s
   c) is characterised by a regular arterial pulse
   d) contraindicates DC cardioversion
   e) may be converted to atrial fibrillation by digoxin.

20. The following are indicated in the treatment of superventricular tachycardia (SVT):
    a) verapamil
    b) carotid sinus massage
    c) nifedipine
    d) digoxin
    e) lignocaine.

21. Pericarditis may occur with:
    a) uraemia
    b) coxsackie B virus
    c) tuberculosis
    d) *Staph. aureus* infection
    e) systemic lupus erythematosus (SLE).

22. Significant stenosis at the origin of the internal carotid artery:
    a) may have no symptoms
    b) can cause ipsilateral hemiplagia
    c) can cause tunnel vision
    d) can cause transient ipsilateral amylobia
    e) always requires carotid endarterectomy.

23. Following a myocardial infarction:
    a) cardiac index (CI) = $2.2 L/mm/m^2$ + hypotension + PCWP = 10 mmHg is compatible with left ventricular failure (LVF)
    b) a left ventricular aneurysm results in persistence of ST segment elevation
    c) beta-blockers reduce mortality
    d) SNP reduces cardiac output.
    e) ACE inhibitors are contraindicated.

24. The following are true of cardiopulmonary resuscitation (CPR):
    a) 40% of patients leave hospital alive
    b) outcome is related to delay in initiation
    c) 'new' CPR increases coronary blood flow
    d) organ perfusion is due to pressure transmitted to great vessels via raised intrathoracic pressure
    e) internal cardiac massage is required in cases of aorbic stenosis.

Answers to multiple-choice questions

1.	a) True;	b) True;	c) False;	d) True;	e) False
2.	a) True;	b) True;	c) True;	d) False;	e) True
3.	a) False;	b) False;	c) False;	d) True;	e) True
4.	a) True;	b) True;	c) True;	d) True;	e) True
5.	a) False;	b) False;	c) False;	d) False;	e) False
6.	a) False;	b) True;	c) False;	d) True;	e) False
7.	a) True;	b) True;	c) False;	d) False;	e) True
8.	a) False;	b) False;	c) False;	d) True;	e) False
9.	a) True;	b) True;	c) True;	d) True;	e) True
10.	a) False;	b) True;	c) True;	d) True;	e) True
11.	a) False;	b) True;	c) False;	d) True;	e) True
12.	a) True;	b) True;	c) True;	d) True;	e) False
13.	a) True;	b) True;	c) True;	d) False;	e) False
14.	a) True;	b) False;	c) True;	d) True;	e) True
15.	a) True;	b) True;	c) True;	d) False;	e) False
16.	a) True;	b) False;	c) True;	d) True;	e) True
17.	a) True;	b) True;	c) True;	d) False;	e) True
18.	a) True;	b) True;	c) True;	d) False;	e) True
19.	a) True;	b) False;	c) True;	d) False;	e) True
20.	a) True;	b) True;	c) False;	d) True;	e) False
21.	a) True;	b) True;	c) True;	d) True;	e) True
22.	a) True;	b) False;	c) False;	d) True;	e) False
23.	a) False;	b) True;	c) True;	d) False;	e) False
24.	a) False;	b) True;	c) True;	d) True;	e) True

SECTION FOUR

THE INTENSIVE CARE UNIT (ICU)

1 Cardiac output

> Discuss the methods by which cardiac output may be assessed in a patient in an intensive care unit.

The standard by which all cardiac output measurement methods have been judged is the *Fick technique*. However, this requires sampling of mixed venous blood and can be performed only when the patient is in a steady state. Measurements of equal accuracy can be obtained by using indicator dilution dye or thermal indicators. Non-invasive estimates of cardiac output may be made using impedance or ultrasound techniques.

Measurement of cardiac output can be by several means:
- *Invasive*
  - indicator dilution
  - thermal indicator dilution.
- *Non-invasive*
  - Doppler ultrasonography
  - thoracic electrical bioimpedance.

Non-invasive methods of measuring cardiac output provide beat-by-beat measurements and so are useful in following rapid changes in stroke output. They are not as accurate as indicator dilution techniques, however.

Indicator dilution

A slug of indicator is injected into the vena cava, the right heart or, preferably, the pulmonary artery. The concentration of the indicator reaching the systemic side of the circulation is plotted against time. The general formula to calculate cardiac output using this technique is:

$$\text{Cardiac output [L/min]} = (60 \times \text{indicator dose [mg]})/(\text{average concentration [mg/L]} \times \text{time [s]})$$

One of the disadvantages of this technique is that recirculation of indicator occurs before the downslope of the curve is complete. A number of techniques have been proposed to overcome the difficulty, but the most commonly used method utilises the exponential character of the downslope.

Of the dyes used for this technique, indocyanine green is the most popular. It is non-toxic and has a relatively short half-life so that repeated measurements can be made.

Indicator dilution curves have also been inscribed using radioactive tracers such as human serum albumin or chromium-labelled red cells.

Thermal indicator dilution

The thermal indicator dilution technique is used routinely in the intensive care situation via a pulmonary artery catheter. The principle of the method is similar to other indicator dilution methods, but the injection and sampling are performed on the right side of the heart. A 10-mL slug of normal saline or 5% dextrose is injected into the right atrium and the temperature change recorded by a thermistor in the pulmonary artery. The dilation curve which results is similar in shape to a dye dilution curve, but there is no recirculation. The calculation is also similar but must be worked out in terms of the 'heat dose'.

Thermal dilution methods have a number of advantages. The indicator is cheap and non-toxic, and repeated measurements may be made without much alteration to the baseline. Arterial puncture and blood withdrawal is not necessary, and the absence of a recirculation curve greatly facilitates measurement of the area under the curve. This becomes particularly important in low-output, high central blood volume states where the recirculation may make dye dilution estimates of output grossly inaccurate.

The disadvantages of this technique are that it requires the passage and correct placement of a special catheter with a thermistor probe which is carefully matched to the processor, and the cost of these devices is not inconsiderable. A further disadvantage is that the bolus is large and mixing with venous blood may be incomplete. In addition, pulmonary arterial flow varies much more with intermittent positive-pressure ventilation (IPPV) than does systemic flow, and there are respiratory fluctuations in temperature in the pulmonary artery. Injection during inspiration may thus give very different results from those obtained with injection during expiration.

Doppler ultrasound

When Doppler ultrasound with a frequency of 1–10 MHz is directed along the long axis of the ascending aorta from a transducer in the suprasternal notch, the sound is reflected back with a frequency shift proportional to the velocity of blood flow. The angle between the direction of blood flow and the ultrasound beam should be kept less than 30 degrees to minimise the error due to lack of alignment. The blood flow velocity curve is integrated to give the average velocity over time, and the stroke volume is then calculated by multiplying the average velocity during each heartbeat by the cross-sectional area of the aorta. Multiplication of stroke volume by heart rate yields cardiac output.

Both continuous and pulsed Doppler systems are in use. The continuous system can measure high velocities but averages the frequency shifts along the whole length of the ascending aorta so that the exact point at which the velocity is measured is unknown. It is therefore difficult to know where to measure the diameter of the aorta. The pulsed Doppler again uses the same transducer to generate and receive the ultrasound but this produces short pulses instead of a continuous stream of ultrasound. The great advantage of the system is that the beam can be focused so that the operator knows the precise depth at which the measurement is being made.

There is a limit to the velocity of blood flow which can be measured since high velocity leads to a large Doppler shift.

There are several disadvantages with measuring cardiac output using Doppler. The aortic diameter must be measured accurately since the cross-sectional area is πr^2. Although aortic diameter can be measured reasonably accurately using echocardiography, the aorta is not completely circular and expands by up to 12% during systole. Furthermore, the site of diameter measurement may not correspond to the position where velocity is measured.

Another source of error of this technique is the shape of the velocity profile. The velocity profile changes shape as it passes through the aortic valve and then through the large diameter of the aorta. Although the central core probably has a velocity close to that in the aortic valve opening, lower velocities may be recorded if the beam is not aligned exactly along the aortic axis.

The measurement of cardiac output via the suprasternal notch is only suitable for intermittent measurements. During anaesthesia better results can be obtained by using a transducer on an oesophageal probe. This is positioned so that it views the descending aorta.

Thoracic electrical bioimpedance

The electrical impedance of a block of tissue fluctuates according to the blood volume contained therein. If two circumferential electrodes are placed around a patient's neck and two around the upper abdomen, a small (<1 mA), constant, high-frequency (>1 kHz) alternating current is passed between the outer electrodes and the resulting potential difference detected by the inner pair. This potential is rectified, smoothed and 'backed off' to yield a zero value. Changes in impedance due to respiration and cardiac activity mark as voltage fluctuations about this zero value.

As respiratory signals are appreciably larger than those due to cardiac activity, measurements are made either with the subject breath-holding, or by using an averaging technique.

Thoracic electrical bioimpedance underestimates cardiac output in septic shock and aortic regurgitation. It is inaccurate when there are intracardiac shunts or arrhythmias. It is, however, fairly accurate and is valuable in the study of rapid changes of cardiac output which could not be followed by other more invasive techniques.

Further reading

Botero M, Lobato EB. Advances in non-invasive cardiac output monitoring: an update. *J Cardiothorac Vasc Anesth* 2001; **15**:631–40.

Dobb GJ, Donovan KD. Non-invasive methods of measuring cardiac output. *Intens Care Med* 1987; **13**:304–9.

Moppett I, Shajar M. Transoesophageal echocardiography. *BJA CEPD Rev* 2001; **1**:72–5.

Muhiudeen IA, Kuecherer HF, Lee E *et al.* Intraoperative estimation of cardiac output by transoesophageal pulsed Doppler echocardiography. *Anesthesiology* 1991; **74**:9–14.

Porter JM, Swain ID. Measurement of cardiac output by electrical impedance plethysmography. *J Biomed Eng* 1987; **9**:222–31.

Thomas AN. Measuring cardiac output. *Curr Anaesth Crit Care* 1996; **6**:309–14.

Wersel RD, Berger RL, Hechtman HB. Current concepts: measurement of cardiac output by thermodilution. *N Engl J Med* 1975; **292**:682–4.

2 Cardiopulmonary resuscitation

Discuss the mechanisms responsible for blood flow during cardiopulmonary resuscitation (CPR).

Blood flow during conventional external cardiac compression is poor. External cardiac massage results in cerebral blood flow of 30–60% of normal and myocardial blood flow of just 5–20% of normal. Lower-limb and visceral blood flow is less than 5% of normal. Flow decreases markedly with time but the relative proportions of flow remain constant.

Pump theories

Two mechanisms have been proposed to explain blood flow during external cardiac compression

- cardiac pump theory
- thoracic pump theory.

In the *cardiac pump theory*, blood is ejected as the cardiac chambers are squeezed between the sternum and spine. Reverse flow is prevented by closure of the mitral and tricuspid valves during chest compression, although valve incompetence has been documented in some studies. It is likely that valve closure is closely related to changes in intrathoracic pressure, and valves may become progressively more incompetent as energy stores within the myocardium are depleted.

The *thoracic pump theory* arose from observations that patients in ventricular fibrillation (VF) can maintain consciousness by repeatedly coughing, suggesting that more complex mechanisms may be involved in generating forward flow. Thoracic compression raises intrathoracic pressure to generate a pressure gradient across the thoracic cavity. Venous valves at the thoracic inlet and within the jugular system together with venous compression prevent retrograde flow. This pressure gradient across the thoracic inlet has been confirmed by catheter studies in humans during CPR, suggesting that the thoracic pump contributes significantly in generating forward flow.

Both mechanisms are probably involved in all forms of cardiac massage, but the degree to which each contributes appears to vary greatly between techniques. As the force of chest compression and chest compliance change during prolonged resuscitation, the dominant mechanism for blood flow may also change. Raised intrathoracic pressure acting through the thoracic pump theory is now thought to contribute significantly in standard CPR, but the cardiac pump theory may contribute more to flow during active compression–decompression (ACD) and other forms of external cardiac massage. Active compression–decompression relies on a suction cup placed over the mid-sternum and compressed to a depth of 3–5 cm with a 50:50 compression–decompression cycle at the standard 80–100 cycles/min. Cohen and associates compared ACD CPR with standard CPR in 62 in-hospital arrests. Twice as many patients who received ACD CPR were resuscitated compared to standard CPR (62% vs 30%).

Mechanisms of forward blood flow during compression are probably similar to those of standard CPR. There is, however, increased left ventricular filling during active decompression, thereby improving venous return, stroke volume and aortic pressures. In contrast to standard CPR, coronary perfusion occurs in both compression and decompression phases of ACD CPR. Active decompression creates a negative intrathoracic pressure that draws a larger volume of blood into the thorax than occurs with standard CPR. Enhanced coronary flow during the compression phase of ACD CPR may be due to an increased blood volume present within the thorax. ACD CPR increased minute ventilation significantly more than standard CPR in human studies through active decompression. This greater chest expansion may then result in a greater rise in intrathoracic pressure within the next compression and thus greater forward flow. Negative intrathoracic pressure during active decompression may be further enhanced by temporarily occluding the endotracheal tube which further enhances venous return. Improved minute ventilation and coronary artery perfusion suggests vital organ perfusion is improved, which may translate into improved long-term survival.

Interposed abdominal compression

Another technique used to improve cardiac output during CPR is interposed abdominal compression. Alternatively the compression between the chest and abdomen is based upon the theory that abdominal compression increases retrograde aortic flow, increases aortic pressure between chest compressions and, thereby, increases coronary blood flow. Abdominal compression also increases intrathoracic pressure by elevating the abdominal contents and diaphragm, increasing central venous pressure. This limits the increase in cerebral perfusion pressure that can be achieved with this technique. Animal and human data are limited for this technique. The incidence of abdominal trauma, regurgitation and other complications are not increased by this technique.

Simultaneous compression/ventilation

Simultaneous compression/ventilation achieves a maximal increase in intrathoracic pressure, thereby increasing cardiac output and cerebral perfusion pressure. However, because there is also an increase in central venous pressure, both cerebral perfusion and coronary perfusion pressure are not enhanced. Intracranial pressure actually increases more than aortic pressure, resulting in decreased cerebral blood flow.

Increasing chest compression

Increasing the force of chest compression increases arterial pressure. However, at compression forces greater than 40 kg, bone and tissue trauma cause a significant increase in the morbidity and mortality. Similarly, high compression rates of up to 150/min increase both cerebral perfusion pressure and cardiac output, but severe internal organ injury has limited the recommended compression rate to 80–100 per minute.

Outlook

The management of CPR continues to be revised with new techniques of external cardiac massage, such as ACD CPR, being evaluated. A better understanding of the mechanisms of blood flow during cardiac massage are emerging through use of transoesophageal echocardiography.

Further reading

Babbs CF, Sack JB, Kern KB. Interposed abdominal compression as an adjunct to cardiopulmonary resuscitation. *Am Heart J* 1994; **127**:412–21.

Baskett PJF. Advances in cardiopulmonary resuscitation. *Br J Anaes* 1992; **69**:182–93.

Berg RA, Kern KB, Saunders AB *et al*. Bystander cardiopulmonary resuscitation: is ventilation necessary? *Circulation* 1993; **88**:1907–15.

Chandra NC, Tsitlik JE, Halperin HT *et al*. Observations of haemodynamics during cardiopulmonary resuscitation. *Crit Care Med* 1990; **18**:929–34.

Cohen TJ, Goldner BG, Maccano PC *et al*. A comparison of active compression–decompression cardiopulmonary resuscitation for cardiac arrests occurring in hospital. *N Eng J Med* 1993; **329**:1918–21.

Criley MJ, Blaufuss AH, Kissel CL. Cough-induced cardiac compression. *J Am Med Assoc* 1976; **236**:1246–50.

Krischer JP, Fine EG, Weisfeldt ML *et al*. Comparison of prehospital conventional and simultaneous compression–ventilation cardiopulmonary resuscitation. *Crit Care Med* 1989; **17**:1263–69.

Pell ACH, Pringle SD, Guly UM *et al*. Assessment of the active compression–decompression device in cardiopulmonary resuscitation using transoesophageal echocardiography. *Resuscitation* 1994; **27**:137–40.

3 Central venous catheter infections

> Discuss the factors associated with venous catheter infections and suggest methods to limit such infections.

The reported incidence of intravascular catheter infection ranges from zero to 100%. The definition of catheter-related infection is imprecise, the clinical presentation is variable, often with few symptoms and signs, and there are difficulties in interpreting the microbiological methods used in diagnosis.

The incidence of infection is influenced by many factors:

- *Patient factors*
  - skin preparation
  - site and position of catheter insertion
  - diameter of blood vessel vs catheter
  - type of insertion (e.g. tunnelled).
- *Medical personnel*
  - hand washing
  - care and technique of insertion
  - subsequent care of insertion site
  - therapy via catheter.
- *Intravascular device*
  - design
  - catheter material, hydrophobicity
  - surface topography of catheter
  - leachable substances from catheter
  - catheter vs vessel diameter
  - flow rate of blood around catheter.

Meticulous aseptic precautions must be taken during insertion of intravascular catheters. This is particularly important in an intensive care unit where patients may be immunocompromised. Cleaning the hands well with soap and water greatly reduces the number of bacteria, but cleaning with 70% ethanol is better. The site of insertion should be cleaned to remove blood, mucus and any other organic debris. A skin preparation such as isopropyl alcohol 70% or iodine 1% in ethanol 70% should be applied and left for an appropriate period to dry before insertion of the catheter.

The longer a device is in place, the more likely the patient is to develop a related infection. It is now widely accepted that plastic peripheral catheters should be removed after 48 hours to reduce the risk of infection. Central catheters can be used for longer if care is taken not to contaminate the catheter and to avoid excessive local trauma during insertion. When appropriate care is

taken there is no correlation between the duration of catheterisation for parenteral nutrition and sepsis. However, there is a correlation between duration of
catheterisation and infection from other types of central catheters. Cannulation
of the subclavian vein has the least risk of infection; cannulation of the femoral
vein has the highest risk.

The widespread use of central catheters with a number of separate lumens
has increased the risk of sepsis. The use of a guidewire to place a new line over
a previous one increases the risk of infection. The incidence is higher for triple-
lumen compared to single-lumen catheters. Tunnelled central lines are less
likely to become colonised and have less chance of related infection.

Its surface characteristics and its composition influence bacterial colonisation of an intravascular device. Coagulase-negative Staphylococci adhere to
microscopic catheter defects on internal and external surfaces and form micro-
colonies. These defects may be scratches, cracks, fissures or even protruding
material. Most plastic catheters are made of synthetic polymers such as polyvi-
nylchloride (PVC), polyethylene, polyurethane and silicone. Bacterial adhesion
is greatest to hydrophobic polymers such as silicone. Bacterial adhesion to polyethylene is greater than to polytetrafluoroethylene (PTFE). Bacterial affinity
for Teflon is less than for either polyethylene or PVC.

Antimicrobial ointments have been applied to the site of insertion.
Polymyxin, neomycin and bacitracin ointment is an example, although it is not
very effective. Contamination of the catheter hub is an important route of
catheter colonisation. It would seem logical to spray the hub regularly with a
topical antiseptic that is active against both fungi and bacteria to block this
route of contamination.

Semi-permeable non-occlusive dressings are useful, as non-permeable
occlusive dressings may increase the local humidity and enhance bacterial
growth. The dressing should not occlude the catheterisation blood vessel
because occlusion encourages thrombus formation and subsequent infection.
Regular changes of intravenous administration sets and dressings have been
proposed to reduce infection. It is thought that infusion sets should be changed
every 24 hours for patients at high risk, such as the severely immunocompromised.

Summary of main approaches to prevention of catheter-related sepsis

Intravascular catheter
1. The smooth surface discourages thrombus formation and microbial colonisation.
2. The fashioned, tapered tip reduces tissue damage on insertion of the catheter.
3. Reduction of leachable substances reduces the inflammatory response.
4. Contained antimicrobials prevent microbial colonisation and infection.

Patient factors

1. Skin preparation can reduce the number of skin micro-organisms and thereby reduce contamination of the catheter at insertion.
2. Use of non-occlusive dressings around the insertion site discourages collection of moisture and microbial multiplication.
3. Application of antiseptics around the insertion site reduces skin microbial colonisation.
4. Regular heparin infusion prevents thrombus formation and subsequent microbial colonisation.

Further reading

Clarke DE, Raffin TA. Infectious complications of indwelling long-term central venous catheters. *Chest* 1990; **97**:966–72 (review).

Decker MD, Edwards KM. Central venous catheter infections. *Pedriatr Clin North Am* 1988; **35**:579–612.

Elliott TSJ. Intravascular device infections. *J Med Microbiol* 1988; **27**:161–7.

Elliott TSJ, D'Abrena VC, Dutton SM. The effect of antibiotics on bacterial colonisation of intravascular devices using a novel in-vitro model. *J Med Microbiol* 1988; **26**:299–35.

Ryan JA, Abel RM, Abbot WM *et al.* Catheter complications in total parenteral nutrition. *N Engl J Med* 1974; **290**:257.

Weightman NC, Simpson EM, Speller DC, Matt MG, Oakhill A. Bacteraemia related to indwelling central venous catheters: prevention, diagnosis and treatment. *Eur J Clin Microbiol Infect Dis* 1988; **7**:125–9.

4 Complications of total parenteral nutrition (TPN)

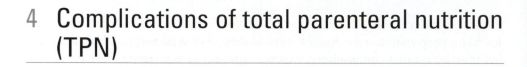

What are the complications of total parenteral nutrition?

Complications of total parenteral nutrition are
- catheter-related sepsis
- catheter occlusions
- metabolic complications
  - refeeding syndrome
  - hepatic dysfunction
  - metabolic bone disease
  - renal dysfunction.

Catheter-related sepsis

Catheter-related sepsis may be confined to the exit site, or infection of the catheter itself may produce fever and bacteraemia. Infection of the catheter is likely if the colony count of blood drawn from the suspected catheter is at least five times greater than a simultaneously drawn peripheral blood sample. Infected catheters should be removed. Routine weekly changes are unnecessary. The femoral route for administration of TPN is associated with a significantly greater incidence of positive tip cultures and bacteraemia compared with arm or neck and shoulder sites.

Catheter occlusions

Central venous catheters may be partially or totally occluded by clot, calcium or lipid deposits. The clot can be treated with urokinase or streptokinase. Blockage by lipid deposits can be prevented and treated using 70% ethyl alcohol as catheter flush. Blockage by calcium deposits may be successfully treated using 0.01 N hydrochloric acid.

Metabolic complications

Rebound hypoglycaemia may occur if a high glucose infusion rate is suddenly discontinued, owing to high levels of endogenous insulin. Hyperglycaemia is the most common metabolic abnormality during parenteral nutrition therapy. Even a modest degree of uncontrolled hyperglycaemia can increase the risk of infection. D-glucose is structurally similar to mannitol and acts as a potent osmotic diuretic in the renal tubules. Hyperosmolar hyperglycaemic non-ketotic dehydration may occur if glucosuria is allowed to develop.

Excessive glucose administration has also been shown to induce *positive sodium and water balance*, increase *circulatory catecholamine levels* and induce *hypophosphataemia*. Hypophosphataemia presents with paraesthesiae, muscular weakness, confusion, convulsions and coma. Plasma phosphate levels may not accurately reflect phosphate deficiency as only 1% is extracellular. Therefore about 10 mmol of phosphate per 1000 kcal of infusate should be provided in TPN solution to prevent deficiency.

Hypercholesterolaemia is the most common alteration of serum lipids. This may be prevented by the use of fat emulsions with a low phospholipid/triglyceride ratio. *Hypertriglyceridaemia* may develop suddenly and appear as 'cloudy serum'. This may be treated by stopping fat administration, infusing heparin to increase plasma lipolytic activity, and infusing glucose with insulin to increase lipoprotein lipase activity in adipose tissue.

Refeeding syndrome is a term used to describe various metabolic abnormalities that can arise as a result of refeeding malnourished patients. It is due to massive cellular uptake of phosphate, potassium and magnesium caused by insulin secretion in response to a glucose load. It may present with a variety of life-threatening clinical manifestations such as arrhythmias, heart failure, respiratory failure, confusion, lethargy, cranial nerve palsy, seizures, haemolysis, thrombocytopenia, fatty liver and sudden death – to name but a few.

The aetiology of *abnormalities in liver function* seen during TPN is obscure and probably multifactorial. Patients on long-term parenteral nutrition may show persistent elevations of liver enzymes, steatosis and cholecystitis, with or without calculi. The use of cyclic infusions and the provision of 30–40% of non-protein calories as fat may minimise the development of parenteral nutrition-related liver dysfunction.

The problem of *low bone mass* measurement in patients on TPN occurs repeatedly and currently does not have an explanation. Similarly, long-term TPN appears to be associated with a decrease in *glomerular filtration rate* (GFR) that is unrelated to underlying disease or nephrotoxic drugs.

Further reading

American Society for Parenteral and Enteral Nutrition (ASPEN) Board of Directors. Guidelines for the use of parenteral and enteral nutrition in adults and paediatric patients. *J Parenter Enteral Nutr* 1993; **17**(suppl. ISA-51SA).

Elia M. Changing concepts of nutrient requirements in disease: implications for artificial nutritional support. *Lancet* 1995; **345**:1279–84.

Hill GL, Windsor JA. Nutritional assessment in clinical practice. *Nutrition* 1995; **11**(suppl. 2):198–201.

Kaye CG, Smith DR. Complications of central venous cannulation. *Br Med J* 1988; **297**:572–73.

Kearney PA, Arnis K. Preoperative nutritional support in critical illness. *Curr Opin Anaesthesiol* 1994; 7:305–9.

Lennard-Jones JE. *A Positive Approach to Nutrition as Treatment*. London: King's Fund Centre, 1992.

Marshal WJ. Perioperative nutritional support. *Care Crit Ill* 1994; **10**:163–7 (review).

McWhirter VP, Pennington CR. Incidence and recognition of malnutrition in hospital. *Br Med J* 1994; **308**:945–8.

Skeie B, Soreide E, Manner T, Askanazi J. Nutrition and breathing. *Care Crit Ill* 1993; **9**:166–9 (review).

5 Enteral versus parenteral feeding

> What are the factors governing the choice between enteral and parenteral feeding for ICU patients?

Advantages of enteral over parenteral feeding are
*   Enteral feeding is cheaper.
*   There is more efficient utilisation of nutrients.
*   It stimulates intestinal blood flow.
*   It maintains the gastrointestinal (GI) mucosal barrier, preventing bacterial translocation and portal endotoxaemia.
*   Disuse atrophy of the GI tract occurs rapidly without enteral feeding.
*   Postoperative enteral feeding reduces septic complications more than the parenteral route.
*   It avoids complications of central venous cannula insertion.
*   It avoids total parenteral nutrition (TPN)-induced immunosupression.
*   There may be greater survival with enteral feeding compared to TPN.

Indications for parenteral nutrition

General
*   Feeding into the GI tract is contraindicated.
*   Enteral feeding fails to meet nutritional requirements and, hence, supplementary TPN is necessary.
*   Enteral access is unobtainable.

Preoperative PN
*   *In mild or moderate malnutrition.* Parenteral nutrition is not normally indicated in patients who need major surgery where there is no delay in operating. It is indicated only if the operation is to be delayed for more than 3–5 days and enteral access or feeding is not possible.
*   *In severe malnutrition.* Preoperative PN is indicated within 1–3 days of admission if immediate surgery is not possible and a substantial period of preoperative starvation is likely.

Postoperative PN
This is indicated in mild to moderate malnutrition where oral or enteral feeding is not expected within 7 days. It should be considered after 5 days in severe malnutrition.

Delivery of PN

Parenteral nutrition can be administered peripherally or centrally. Peripheral parenteral nutrition (PPN) is usually administered via a forearm vein. The rationale for using the peripheral route is that the majority of patients with temporary intestinal failure requiring TPN do so for less than 14 days. The development of peripheral vein thrombophlebitis is a troublesome complication which often interferes with successful PPN. Its development may be delayed by using non-irritant fine-bore polyurethane or silicone elastomer catheters sited in a large vein in the forearm. TPN support via the central route is necessary when parenteral feeding is indicated for longer than 2 weeks, peripheral venous access is limited, osmolality of the infusated is high due to nutrient needs of fluid restriction, and the benefits of TPN outweigh the risks.

6 Assessment of nutritional status

> How would you assess a patient's nutritional status and nutritional requirements in the ICU?

There has been much debate about the best method to determine calorie needs in the hospitalised patient.

Resting energy expenditure

The total daily energy expenditure can be estimated by calculating the resting energy expenditure (REE), which is defined as the amount of energy required to maintain basic metabolic function in the resting state. The REE can be calculated using the Harris–Benedict equation:

$$REE \text{ (males)} = 66.5 + (13.7 \times \text{bodyweight}) + (5.0 \times \text{height}) \, (6.8 \times \text{age})$$
$$REE \text{ (females)} = 65.5 + (9.6 \times \text{bodyweight}) + (1.7 \times \text{height}) \, (4.7 \times \text{age})$$
where height is in centimetres, bodyweight is in kilograms and age is in years.

The REE is then multiplied by a stress factor to allow for the effects of disease (i.e. sepsis or burns) on energy expenditure. This figure is finally multiplied by an 'activity factor' which takes into account the energy requirements of normal or reduced activity.

Disease has an unpredictable effect on energy expenditure and it is clearly better to measure REE by indirect calorimetry using the open-circuit vented hood system, rather than estimate it. This is the most common method of measuring energy expenditure and it is based on the measurement of oxygen consumption and carbon dioxide production. It may be difficult to extrapolate this short period of measurement to a 24-hour period, and even if available it is not always practicable owing to the stringent conditions necessary for its measurement.

Most hospitalised patients require 25–30 kcal/kg per day. Those requiring mechanical ventilation lie in the lower end of this range. In a septic, catabolic patient who is having TPN for an average of 2 weeks, a caloric intake of 80% of requirements is usually appropriate. Patients with burns or trauma may require 40–45 kcal/kg per day. The provision of excess calories is harmful and should be avoided.

Protein intake

Nitrogen is utilised as a marker for protein intake. One gram of nitrogen is equivalent to 6.25 g of protein. The estimation of protein requirements may be performed in various ways:

- nitrogen balance
- non-protein calorie to nitrogen ratio
- based on bodyweight.

Nitrogen balance is a relative index subject to technical and collection errors:

$$\text{Nitrogen balance} = (\text{protein intake [g]}/6.25) - (\text{urinary nitrogen [g]} + 4)$$

where 4 is the empirical and often imprecise factor added to account for non-urinary nitrogen losses that occur in faeces and sweat.

A non-protein calorie to nitrogen ratio is often used with a range of 100–200 kcal/g of nitrogen in critically ill patients.

Protein requirement may also be assessed based on bodyweight. Utilisation of exogenous protein for purposes of anabolism levels off at about 1.5 g/kg per day, and no benefit is seen at levels above this except for patients with large burns who lose considerable amounts of protein from the burn site.

In practice, achieving a positive nitrogen balance in critically ill catabolic patients may prove difficult. Current commercially available amino acid solutions for parenteral use may not reflect the pattern of loss of amino acids released from the skeletal muscles of a critically ill patient.

Glucose

Glucose provides 3.4 kcal/g when used as an energy source for parenteral nutrition. Administration of carbohydrates will stimulate the secretion of insulin which has anabolic effects such as increasing the uptake of glucose into tissues, inhibiting lipolysis and protein breakdown and stimulating protein synthesis by increasing amino acid uptake into cells. The daily adult intake requirement of glucose is about 4–5 g/kg per day in severely catabolic patients.

Lipids

Fat emulsions are commercially prepared from soyabean or sunflower oils in concentrations of 10% and 20% which provide 1.1 kcal/mL and 2.0 kcal/mL respectively. Lipids prevent essential fatty acid deficiency when they form at least 3% of total daily calorific requirements. Lipid requirements are about 1–1.5 g/kg per day.

Non-protein calories are provided as a mixture of carbohydrate and fat in a ratio of approximately 70:30. Provision of additional calories as fat rather than as glucose may be advantageous for patients actively weaning from mechanical ventilation. However, excess fat administration has been associated with hyperlipidaemia, hypoxia due to impairment of pulmonary function, an increased rate of infection due to depression of humoral and cell-mediated immunity, and a higher postoperative mortality rate.

Minerals and micronutrients

Provision of adequate amounts of sodium, potassium, calcium, magnesium and phosphate is usually guided by serial estimation of plasma levels.

Micronutrients include two main classes of substances required in small amounts, the inorganic trace elements and organic vitamins. They play a key role as cofactors or coenzymes in enzymatic reactions that take place in intermediary metabolism and thus play a vital role in key metabolic processes.

Micronutrients also form part of the free-radical scavenging system which prevents damage to the polyunsaturated fatty acid component of cells and intracellular organelles. Supplementation in excess of requirements may be harmful as certain micronutrients such as vitamins A and D have a narrow margin of toxicity. Examples of other micronutrients are zinc, copper, selenium, manganese, chromium and molybdenum.

7 Hypothermia

> A 65-year-old woman is admitted unconscious with a temperature of 20°C. How
> should she be managed?

Effects of hypothermia

CVS
- Decreased cardiac output below 32°C with bradycardia and reduced MAP.
- Vasoconstriction below 32°C, increasing afterload and thus myocardial work.
- ECG changes including widening QRS complex and increased PR interval, prolonged QT interval and J waves. Risk of ventricular fibrillation (VF) below 28°C.
- Increased blood viscosity, which increases myocardial work.

Respiratory
- Decreased CO_2 production.
- Increased anatomical and physiological dead-space.
- Diaphragm fatigue.
- Metabolic acidosis, causing pulmonary hypertension.

Gastrointestinal system
- Decreased hepatic and renal blood flow.
- Decreased liver metabolism.

Metabolism
- Decrease in metabolic rate by 8% per °C.
- Shivering increases O_2 consumption by up to 800%. Resultant increased muscle flow may accelerate heat loss.
- Hypothermia shifts O_2 dissociation curve to the left, reducing O_2 delivery.
- Increased stress response.
- Hyperglycaemia secondary to increased glycogenolysis and reduced insulin production.
- Reduced drug metabolism.

CNS
- CNS protection below 24°C.
- Pupils fixed and dilated below 30°C.

Other effects
- Increased bleeding time of skin, increased prothrombin time (PT) and partial thromboplastin time (PTT).

- Decreased platelet count and white cell count.
- Increased risk of DVT and PE.
- Immunosuppression.

Renal
- GFR is reduced below a core temperature of 20°C.

Management of the hypothermic patient

The management of this patient should involve a team approach for prioritising life-threatening injury and a system of sequential review so that little is overlooked. The advanced trauma life support (ATLS) provides a common language.

Primary survey

The airway is obtained, protected and secured. In a patient with a body temperature of 20°C this will involve endotracheal intubation. If anaesthesia is employed, cricoid pressure should be utilised. It should be assumed that the patient has cervical spinal injury until disproven. The neck is immobilised in a hand cervical collar. Sandbags are placed on each side of the head and the neck, and the forehead is firmly taped to both sides of the trolley. In-line stabilisation of the neck during laryngoscopy and intubation is an acceptable alternative to the hand collar.

The patient's lungs are ventilated with 100% oxygen. Adequate and symmetrical breathing on both sides of the chest is assessed and mechanical dysfunction such as pneumo/haemothorax; major airway damage or airway obstruction is sought.

The circulation is assessed. Pulses are checked, blood response recorded and two large-bore intravenous cannulae are sited and fluid resuscitation commenced. The cardiac rhythm is recorded.

With ABC established, the patient is assessed for neurological damage. Evidence of brain and spinal injury is specifically sought. The patient is exposed to allow full assessment. The back is examined during this phase, and logrolling is required to prevent spinal cord injury. Hidden, untreated injuries may be lethal.

This patient with a core temperature of 20°C will have a depressed cardiovascular system. There is a likelihood of VF at this temperature as well as bradycardia and increased afterload due to vasoconstriction. Basic life support should be commenced during the primary survey if there is no cardiac output. The arrhythmia should be treated according to Resuscitation Council UK guidelines.

Secondary survey

Once the primary survey is complete a systemic examination of the patient during the secondary survey follows. Chest, pelvic and lateral neck x-rays are required during this phase. During the secondary survey steps should be taken to rewarm the patient. These steps include the following:

1. Monitor core temperature with an oesophageal temperature probe placed behind the heart.
2. All fluids, both colloid and crystalloid, should be warmed to 37°C prior to infusion.
3. Inhaled gases are warmed by humidifiers to 40°C.
4. All exposed parts (including the head) should be covered. A heating blanket should be placed over the patient.
5. More invasive but very effective treatment is intraperitoneal irrigation with saline warmed to 37°C.
6. Patients should be slowly rewarmed and cardiac life support continued until the patient's core temperature is 37°C.

There is CNS protection at temperatures below 24°C, with pupils being fixed and dilated below 30°C.

Further reading

American College of Surgeons. *ATLS: Advanced Trauma Life Support*. Chicago: ACS.

Driscoll PA, Vincent CA. Organising an efficient trauma team. *Injury* 1992; **23**:107–10.

Hessel EA, Schmer G, Dilliard DH. Platelet kinetics during deep hypothermia. *J Surg Res* 1980; **28**:23–9.

Luna C, Maier RV, Pavlin EG *et al*. Incidence and hypothermia in seriously injured patients. *J Trauma* 1987; **27**:1014–18.

Pickering BG, Bristow GK, Craig DB. Core rewarming by peritoneal irrigation in accidental hypothermia with cardiac arrest. *Anaesth Analges* 1977; **56**:574–7.

8 Trauma to chest

> **What problems may occur in the intensive care therapy unit in a victim of severe blunt trauma to the chest, and how may these problems be managed?**

High-energy accidents frequently result in chest or abdominal trauma. These injuries carry a significant mortality which may be reduced by early, decisive intervention.

Severe chest injury may involve any structure within the thoracic cavity. Hypoxia is a common and dangerous feature, often combined with hypertension secondary to large-volume haemorrhage within the thorax. Hyperventilation, with concomitant hypercarbia, is not infrequently seen; its presence implies severe chest injury.

Airway, breathing and circulation (ABC) are assessed and secured initially. Exposure of the patient allows a thorough evaluation for additional injuries. A clear airway must be ensured and a high inspired oxygen concentration delivered. The assessment of breathing includes elucidation of:
- the pattern and rate of spontaneous ventilation
- abnormalities of chest wall movement
- equality of breath sounds
- alteration in resonance to percussion
- signs of external injury such as bruising or penetrating wounds.
  Life-threatening chest injuries are:
- pneumothorax
- haemothorax
- pericardial tamponade
- pulmonary contusion
- myocardial contusion
- flail chest
- great vessel disruption
- tracheobronchial disruption
- diaphragmatic rupture
- cardiac rupture.

The circulation is often markedly impaired and management consists of rapid transfusion of fluid via large-bore intravenous access. The majority of patients with penetrating chest wounds have a haemopneumothorax. A tension pneumothorax should be diagnosed and managed on clinical grounds, and its management should not wait for radiological confirmation. The entire blood volume may be contained within the thoracic cavity so that the presence of a demonstrative haemothorax means major haemorrhage. Massive haemothorax should be managed by chest drain insertion and simultaneous restoration of circulating blood volume. Initial drainage of 1000 ml of blood after insertion of the chest drain, or drainage of 1500 mL in the first 24 hours following insertion, may prompt exploratory thoracotomy.

Flail chest describes the presence of multiple rib fractures where there is paradoxical movement of the chest wall during respiration. The resultant hypoxaemia is due to contusion and subsequent shunting of blood through the underlying lung. Multiple rib fractures are extremely painful and hyperventilation is frequently seen. Management involves:

- provision of supplemental oxygen
- careful fluid resuscitation to avoid iatrogenic oedema of the contused lung
- analgesia.

Ideally, regional anaesthesia should be used as this provides high-quality analgesia and allows restoration of ventilation. Thoracic epidural analgesia is extremely effective and is best sited at the vertebral level of the chest injury. Bupivacaine 0.125% usually provides excellent analgesia. Addition of an opioid may further improve ventilatory function. Alternative techniques include paravertebral analgesia and intercostal nerve blockade. Intrapleural administration of local anaesthetic has been shown to be effective and can be accomplished by introducing 50 mL of 0.1% bupivacaine via the chest drain.

Potent opioids administered intravenously may provide effective analgesia, but may also exacerbate hypoventilation and cough suppression. Non-steroidal anti-inflammatory drugs work well in combination with opioids, if not contraindicated.

High-quality analgesia is vital because patients with painful, bony chest injury tend to hypoventilate and cough inadequately. They are at risk of hypercarbia, hypoxia, atelectasis, sputum retention and pneumonia.

Both blunt and penetrating injuries to the chest may result in pericardial tamponade resulting in hypertension resistant to fluid administration, muffled heart sounds, small complex ECG, and elevated jugular venous pressure. Tamponade should be managed by needle pericardiocentesis with continuous ECG monitoring.

Great thoracic vessel disruption is frequently fatal and may develop after the initial injury. Thoracic aortic disruption may present with chest or back pain, hypertension and loss of one or both radial pulses; it may be diagnosed by widening of the mediastinum on chest x-ray. A thoracic computed tomography scan or an arch aortogram may be diagnostic. Prompt diagnosis and emergency thoracotomy may be life-saving, requiring surgical correction and possible cardiopulmonary bypass.

Tracheobronchial injuries are uncommon but life-threatening. They frequently present as hypoxaemia, haemoptysis and hypertension and require surgical correction. Haemopneumothorax is usually present. Endotracheal or endobronchial tube placement may be best accomplished under direct vision using a rigid or fibreoptic bronchoscope.

Chest-injured patients require management in an ICU or high-dependency area for all but the simplest injuries. The emphasis of therapy for severe chest injuries has shifted from an invasive approach to one of careful monitoring and provision of potent analgesia. This may allow the avoidance of mechanical ventilation in the patient whose ventilation, alveolar expansion and sputum clearance are inhibited by the pain of rib fractures. Mechanical ventilation should be used in resistantly hypoxaemic patients. Other indications for endotracheal intubation in patients with severe chest injury include unconsciousness, inability to maintain an adequate airway, and severe hypoventilation and hypercarbia.

It is very occasionally useful to provide differential lung ventilation. This is achieved via an endbronchial double-lumen tube. It is indicated when the two lungs have markedly different requirements for positive end-expiratory pressure (PEEP) and inspiratory and expiratory times and the pulmonary shunt is predominantly unilateral. Jet ventilation has been shown to be effective in managing these patients, allowing adequate carbon dioxide elimination while generating very low peak and mean airway pressures.

Blunt injury to the anterior chest wall may result in myocardial contusion. ECG monitoring should be used in all patients. Arrhythmias, typically ventricular extrasystoles, or more rarely fibrillation, are frequently seen. Lignocaine 1 mg/kg may help prevent the occurrence of arrhythmias.

Injuries to the lower chest may damage intra-abdominal structures such as the spleen, liver or kidneys. Surgical assessment of the abdomen is urgently required if there is abdominal tenderness, rigidity, bruising, distension or persistent hypovolaemia. Similarly, pelvic injury and cervical spine injury must be excluded. A hard collar should be kept on the patient until the cervical spine has been cleared.

Further reading

Hillman KM, Barber JD. Asychronous independent lung ventilation (AILV). *Crit Care Med* 1980; 8:390–5.

Kish G, Kozloff L, Joseph WL, Adkins PC. Indications for early thoracotomy in the management of chest trauma. *Ann Thorac Surg* 1976; **22**:22–8.

Kram HB, Wohlmuth DA, Appel PL, Shoemaker W. Clinical and radiological indications for arteriography in blunt chest trauma. *J Vasc Surg* 1987; 6:168–75.

Mackersie RC, Shackford SR, Hoyt DB, Karagianes TG. Continuous epidural fentanyl analgesia: ventilatory function improvement with routine use in treatment of blunt chest injury. *J Trauma* 1987; **27**:1207–12.

O'Kelly E, Garry B. Continuous pain relief for multiple fractured ribs. *Br J Anaesth* 1981; **53**:989–91.

Rocco A, Reiestad F, Gudman J, McKay W. Intrapleural administration of local anaesthetics for pain relief in patients with multiple rib fractures. *Reg Anaesth* 1987; **12**:10–14.

9 Transfer between hospitals

Assess the problems of transfer of critically ill patients between hospitals.

Transfer of critically ill patients is indicated if there is a need for additional care not available at the patient's current location. Recommendations of the Intensive Care Society and the British Paediatric Association to centralise intensive care services in regional units will make inter-hospital transfer more common. There is evidence that the number of adult transfers between general, neurosurgical and cardiac units in the UK exceeds 11 000 per annum.

Potential problems are:

- an unstable patient
- the isolated environment during transfer
- limited equipment
- the difficulty or impossibility of treatment in a moving vehicle
- the safety of personnel.

Prior to transfer the patient must be resuscitated and stabilised as far as possible. Some patients may require specific therapy prior to transfer. A patient with multiple injuries may require a laporotomy to control intra-abdominal haemorrhage prior to transfer to a neurosurgical centre for head injury. Early communication with the receiving hospital is vital to agree on mode and expectation of transfer. The safest and easiest means of controlling the airway in critically ill patients is tracheal intubation with controlled ventilation facilitated by sedation and analgesia. Documentation and any cross-matched blood should be taken with the patient. A journey should not be started with an unstable patient because of the high risk of complications during the journey.

There are four categories of adult inter-hospital transfer:

- *Category 1* – for upgrade of care requiring specialist support or investigation (e.g. burns, cardiothoracic, liver, neurosurgery, paediatric)
- *Category 2* – for upgrade of care where a particular type of organ support is not available locally (e.g. renal replacement therapy)
- *Category 3* – where a patient is moved nearer to home
- *Category 4* – due to a local lack of available critical-care beds.

In the isolated environment during a transfer it is vital to have both a doctor and a nurse with experience in assessing and managing seriously injured patients. Anaesthetic skills are particularly valuable for airway care and for sophisticated monitoring during the journey. An anaesthetist must escort every intubated and ventilated patient. Delegation to non-anaesthetists or junior trainees is inappropriate. The doctor and nurse are professionally responsible for the patient during transfer and must be well informed about the patient before the journey starts. Ideally they should have been involved in the initial patient resuscitation.

Guidelines for anaesthetic monitoring apply equally to patients undergoing transfer as they do in the anaesthetic room. Relying on clinical signs and symptoms is unacceptable. The ECG should be monitored continuously as should the blood pressure. Invasive blood pressure monitoring is desirable in unstable patients. All lines must be secured and arterial and central venous lines should be clearly labelled to prevent inadvertent drug injection through them. Patients quickly become cold in an ambulance and hence should be kept warm with blankets or preferably a space blanket. Pulse oximeters may be unreliable owing to movement artefacts or peripheral vasoconstriction. Monitors themselves should be robust, compact and have easily readable displays and an adequate power supply. Information displayed by the monitors must be carefully recorded. Ideally monitors should print out a hard copy displaying trends. All monitoring and other equipment used for patient transfer should be regularly serviced, disposables replaced and drugs regularly checked for expiry date and replaced when used.

Ventilators, oxygen supplies and airway equipment should be checked prior to departure. The volume of oxygen required for the transfer should be calculated and a generous safety margin should be allowed to cater for ambulance diversion or breakdown. The oxygen supply can fail and a self-inflating bag should be available. Therapy should be simplified wherever possible.

Gravity-dependent infusion devices are unreliable during transfer and electronic infusion pumps should be used with an adequate power supply. The ambulance should carry a range of airway equipment to allow reintubation if necessary. Similarly a range of intravenous cannulae as well as crystalloid and colloid infusion fluids should be carried. Cardiac resuscitation drugs, sedatives, analgesics and muscle relaxants should be available during transfer.

The ambulance rarely needs to travel at great speed, which can worsen cardiovascular instability. A smooth ride at constant speed is safer. The patient should be placed in the ambulance head first so as better to tolerate any sudden deceleration during the journey. If life-saving procedures like endotracheal intubation have to be carried out along the way it is more sensible to stop the ambulance briefly, because assessment and treatment are almost impossible in a moving ambulance.

Air transfer may be by helicopter, fixed-wing aircraft or commercial liner. Specific problems with air transportation are a decrease in available oxygen in unpressurised cabins at altitude; hence the need for higher inspired oxygen tensions. Pressurised aircraft are pressurised only to an equivalent of 6000 feet above sea level. Thus added oxygen is almost always necessary in the critically ill. Gas-containing spaces such as pneumothoraces, bowel and tracheal tube cuffs expand during ascent as ambient pressure drops. A pneumothorax should be drained prior to transfer by air.

The referring hospital must carry adequate insurance for injuries sustained by the escorts and patients on the way to the specialist centre. The ambulance is purely an extension of their hospital.

The escorts must be able to give the specialist centre an accurate description of all injuries, interventions since admission and any drugs and intravenous fluids given. They should not leave until they have done so. All medical notes and nursing clinical notes, observation charts, drug prescription sheets and x-ray films and scans should be left with the receiving team.

Further reading

Association of Anaesthetists of Great Britain and Ireland. *Recommendations for Standards of Monitoring during Anaesthesia and Recovery*. London: AA, 1988.

Bion JF, Wilson IH, Taylor PA. Transporting critically ill patients by ambulance: audit by sickness scoring. *Br Med J* 1988; **296**:170.

Gentleman D, Dearden M, Midgley S, Maclean D. Guidelines for the resuscitation and transfer of patients with serious head injury. *Br Med J* 1993; **307**:547–52.

Intensive Care Society. *Guidelines for Transport of the Critically Ill Adult*. London: ICS, 1997.

Lambert SM, Willett K. Transfer of multiply injured patients for neurosurgical opinion: a study of the adequacy of assessment and resuscitation. *Injury* 1993; **24**:333–6.

Oakley PA. The need for standards for inter-hospital transfer. *Anaesthesia* 1994; **49**:563–6.

Rose J, Valtoren S, Jennett B. Avoidable factors contributing to death after injury. *Br Med J* 1977; **ii**:615–8.

Wallace PGM, Ridley SA. ABC of intensive care: transport of critically ill patients. *Br Med J* 1999; **319**:368–71.

10 Metabolic requirements

> How may metabolic requirements of a patient needing total parenteral nutrition be assessed?

Assessment of the nutritional status of a patient provides information about the degree and type of nutritional depletion and assesses the need for nutritional support. Malnutrition adversely affects immunity and the function of skeletal, cardiac and respiratory muscles. This may lead to a reduction in mobility, delayed recovery and predisposition to thromboembolism and death.

There is growing evidence to suggest that starting nutrition within 24 hours of major surgery, injury or burn is ideal.

A detailed history and thorough clinical examination of the patient is the most important technique for nutritional assessment. Measurement of hand-grip strength, plasma proteins and electromyography studies of muscle function supplement the findings from a history and a physical examination.

Enteral feeding requires at least 25 cm of ileum. Paralytic ileus affects only the stomach and colon so that small bowel motility and absorption often remain normal. Thus bowel sounds and flatus are *not* required to start enteral feeding. Early enteral feeding through a nasojejunal tube or feeding jejunostomy may prevent paralytic ileus.

Traditional methods of nutritional assessment

Weight loss
Weight loss from the ideal or usual weight is a useful predictor of complications, especially if hypoalbuminaemia is also present.

Anthropometry
Triceps skin-fold thickness (TSF) is useful in serial measurements or as part of a general assessment. The creatinine–height index is also used.

Immune competence
Non-specific indicators are total lymphocyte count and delayed hypersensitivity tests.

Plasma proteins
Albumin is useful as a predictor when associated with other changes (e.g weight loss), but is also affected by primary disease and extracellular water shifts. Other plasma proteins are prealbumin, transferrin and retinol-binding protein.

Prognostic nutritional index (PNI)
This is based on a formula involving albumin, transferrin, TSF and delayed hypersensitivity tests.

Tests of muscle function
* Hand-grip strength (<85% of normal) is a useful predictor of postoperative complications but is of limited use in the critically ill.
* Electromyographic abnormalities are specific for malnutrition and correlate with surgical outcome.

Subjective goal assessment (SGA)
SGA is a method that is accurate and consistent. It covers:
1. *History* – weight change, dietary change, GI symptoms >2 weeks, functional capacity underlying disease, effect on metabolic stress.
2. *Physical factors* – loss of subcutaneous fat, muscle wasting, ankle or sacral oedema, ascites.

Bedside nutritional assessment
This consists of:
1. *Protein and energy balance* – compare dietary history with rate of weight loss.
2. *Body composition* – weight loss from usual weight, palpation of skin folds and bony prominence of scapula for fat and protein loss respectively.
3. *Physiological function* – history of a change in exercise tolerance or wound healing, with bedside tests for grip strength and respiratory muscle function.
4. *Evidence of metabolic stress* – major trauma or surgery <1 week, sepsis or inflammation.

Further reading
McWhirter JP, Pennington CR. Incidence and recognition of malnutrition in hospital. *Br Med J* 1994; **308**:945–8.
Uehara M, Plank LD, Hill GL. Components of energy expenditure in patients with severe sepsis and major trauma: a basis for clinical care. *Crit Care Med* 1999; **27**:1295–302.

11 Nitric oxide use

Discuss the therapeutic role of nitric oxide in intensive care.

Nitric oxide (NO) is produced from the terminal guanidino nitrogen of the semi-essential amino acid L-arginine, during its conversion to L-citrulline, a reaction catalysed by a family of nitric oxide syntheses (NOS). These are complex haemoproteins with similarities to cytochrome P-450 reductase.

NO exerts its physiological role by binding to the haem moiety of intracellular guanylate cyclase. This produces a conformational change in the enzyme, increasing production of cyclic guanosine 3,5,-monophosphate (cGMP). This increase in cGMP produces smooth muscle relaxation by a mechanism that is still not fully understood.

Inhibitory non-adrenergic non-cholinergic nerves are the only neural bronchodilator pathways in human airways. It is thought that the neurotransmitter is NO released during depolarisation of the peripheral nerve ending. NO then diffuses into the underlying bronchial smooth muscle.

NO is probably also involved in neuronal vasodilator mechanisms in the pulmonary circulation. It is likely that adenosine triphosphate (ATP) released by sympathetic nerves causes the release of NO from endothelial cells which diffuses into the vessel wall muscle producing relaxation. NO-mediated neurotransmission may therefore act to counter processes which would lead to increased vascular and bronchial tone.

NO may act to modify the effects of artificially induced bronchoconstriction, rather than to produce a reduction in resting bronchial tone. NO inhalation by normal individuals does not produce a change in airway resistance, but in asthmatic subjects it produces a small but variable reduction. Nitrovasodilators, such as sodium nitroprusside and glyceryl trinitrate, which produce a local release of NO, also relax airway smooth muscle.

There is a tonic production of NO in the pulmonary circulation and hypoxia reduces this release. There is thus a mechanism which links hypoxia to a reduction in baseline vasodilator tone. This may contribute to the phenomenon known as 'hypoxic pulmonary vasoconstriction', crucial to the matching of ventilation and perfusion (V–Q).

Severe sepsis and other inflammatory states produce widespread and uncontrolled release of NO. This contributes to the vascular hyperactivity so characteristic of these conditions and leads to systemic hypertension.

The acute respiratory distress syndrome (ARDS) represents the pulmonary manifestation of a global inflammatory process. ARDS produces patchy pulmonary collapse and consolidation, and the deficit in gas exchange is produced principally by impaired V–Q matching and hypoxic pulmonary vasoconstriction. The uncontrolled release of vasodilating NO would undoubtedly contribute to this. In addition to a loss of local vascular regulation, vasoconstriction and mechanical blockage of vessels occurs, leading to a reduction in cross-sectional area of the pulmonary vasculature. This results in pulmonary hypertension, which may be severe enough to produce right heart failure. In ARDS the delivery of a vasodilator via the inhaled route has an attractive logic. The dilator would only be delivered to lung units in continuity with ventilating gas, and would therefore produce a recruitment of blood flow to ventilated alveoli. A short half-life ensures that systemic side-effects are unlikely, as the drug would not reach the systemic circulation.

This theoretical approach has been shown to work in practice, with a number of studies of inhaled NO (in concentrations from 0.5 to 32 parts per million) demonstrating useful and sustained improvements in oxygenation and pulmonary haemodynamics. However, no study has yet demonstrated a clear reduction in mortality or morbidity. This may reflect the fact that mortality in ARDS is intimately related to underlying disease as well as respiratory failure, or that there are toxicity issues yet to be identified. Additionally, there are considerable technical and logistical difficulties to overcome in accurately and safely administering inhaled NO.

The inhalation of NO may cause toxicity via a number of routes. NO combines with oxygen to produce toxic nitric dioxide (NO_2) under conditions of high oxygen concentration. NO_2 levels in inhaled gas must therefore be measured. Under certain conditions, NO combines with the superoxide radical to produce the highly toxic peroxynitrite ion which is cytotoxic and harmful to surfactants, lipids, nucleic acids and proteins. Inflamed lungs are likely to produce superoxide and hence peroxynitrite. Only the vaguest ideas exist about the conditions prevailing in an inflamed lung receiving high concentrations of inspired oxygen. In addition, the nitrite produced as an end metabolite of NO will produce methaemoglobinaemia, which can reach concentrations sufficient to significantly impair the oxygen-carrying capacity of the blood.

Current clinical research centres on the role of NO in normal pulmonary physiology, the vascular collapse of severe sepsis and in the manipulation of the pulmonary circulation in ARDS. In spite of huge research efforts little knowledge has been translated into clearly efficacious therapies.

Further reading

Cuthbertson BH, Dellinger P, Dyar OJ et al. UK guidelines for the use of inhaled nitric oxide therapy in adult ICUs. American–European Consensus Conference on ALI/ARDS. *Intensive Care Med* 1997; **23**:1212–18.

Dupry RM, Shore SA, Drazen JM et al. Broncho-dilator action of inhaled nitric oxide in guinea pigs. *J Clin Invest* 1992; **90**:421–8.

Gerlach H, Pappert D, Lewandowski K, Rossaint R, Falke KJ. Long-term inhalation with evaluated low doses of nitric oxide for selective improvement of
oxygenation in patients with adult respiratory distress syndrome. *Int Care
Med* 1993; **19**:443–9.

Palmer RMJ, Ferrige AC, Moncada S. Nitric oxide release accounts for the bio-
logical activity of endothelium-derived relaxing factor. *Nature* 1987;
327:524–6.

Puybasset L, Rouby JJ, Mourgeon E *et al.* Inhaled nitric oxide in acute respiratory failure: dose–response curves. *Int Care Med* 1994; **20**:319–27.

Quinn AC, Petros A, Vallance P. Nitric oxide: an endogenous gas. *Br J Anaesth*
1995; **74**:443–51.

Vallance P, Collier J. Biology and clinical relevance of nitric oxide. *Br Med J*
1994; **309**:453–7.

12 Positive end-expiratory pressure (PEEP)

> Discuss the use of positive end-expiratory pressure in patients requiring mechanical ventilation. What problems may arise from the use of PEEP?

Positive end-expiratory pressure is the maintenance of a positive pressure within the lungs throughout expiration, and may be applied during intermittent positive-pressure ventilation (IPPV) or during spontaneous breathing – when it is called 'continuous positive airway pressure' (CPAP). There are advantages and disadvantages to PEEP:

- **Advantages**
  - increased airway pressure
  - increased functional residual capacity (FRC)
  - recruitment of collapsed alveoli
  - decreased airway resistance
  - reduced V–Q mismatch
  - improved distribution of inspired gas
  - reduced work of breathing
  - increased P_{O_2} due to increase in FRC
  - prevention of surfactant aggregation, reducing alveolar collapse.

- **Disadvantages**
  - impaired CO_2 elimination
  - reduced cardiac output
  - reduced glomerular filtration rate
  - increased pulmonary vascular resistance
  - decreased flow in West's zone 1, causing increased dead-space.

Discussion

A number of mechanisms have been suggested for the improvement in gas exchange seen generally with the use of PEEP and CPAP. The most likely is the restoration of FRC towards normal, increasing it above the closing capacity and recruiting previously collapsed alveoli. The work of breathing is reduced, decreasing oxygen consumption and alleviating respiratory muscle fatigue. Other effects may be the prevention of surfactant aggregation associated normally with the use of large tidal volumes; and the enhancement of the lung's ability to degrade bradykinin and reduction of protein flux into the alveoli by increasing the alveolar P_{O_2}. A prophylactic role in preventing acute respiratory distress syndrome (ARDS) by conserving surfactant and the facilitation of weaning of patients with chronic obstructive airway disease has been claimed. CPAP has been used for many years in the management of respiratory distress in infants and to facilitate weaning from mechanical ventilation of adults whose oxygenation is dependent on PEEP. The splinting effect of CPAP on the upper respiratory tract airway has also been used in the treatment of obstructive sleep apnoea.

The therapeutic benefits of PEEP must be balanced against the unwanted side-effects. Excessive PEEP or CPAP reduces cardiac output by decreasing left ventricular wall compliance by dilation of the right ventricle consequent to an increase in pulmonary vascular resistance. Left ventricular function may be impaired directly by the external pressure exerted by the forced expansion of the lungs. Thus, while the arterial oxygenation may be improved, oxygen delivery may be diminished. A particular problem may occur in patients with a right to left intracardiac shunt, which may be worsened with the increased PVR. Overdistension of 'normal' alveoli may occur in patients with non-uniform lung disease.

The resultant diversion of pulmonary blood flow to unventilated lung may worsen oxygenation. This effect may be seen during one-lung anaesthesia if PEEP is applied to the dependent, ventilated lung. PEEP of $5-10\,cmH_2O$ is commonly used. A more controversial application is the use of PEEP at levels up to $40\,cmH_2O$ in selected cases of ARDS or asthma. PEEP reduces urine output secondary to a decrease in renal cortical perfusion and increased secretion of ADH. The mechanism for these changes in renal function is probably the effective reduction in intravascular volume and reduction in renal perfusion pressure associated with PEEP. Cortical renal blood flow may also be reduced by redistribution within the kidney secondary to increased renal venous pressures.

The increased alveolar pressure produced by PEEP exerts a direct effect on pulmonary capillary resistance by reducing transmural pressure gradient. This is important in zones 1 and 2 where alveolar pressure exceeds venous pressure. As the alveoli expand, the tethering of the larger vessels to the surrounding connective tissue may cause them to increase in calibre. However, the smaller vessels tend to collapse as they are stretched by increasing alveolar distension, and a net increase in vascular resistance results.

PEEP increases the production of antidiuretic hormone (ADH) which is accompanied by an increase in the plasma concentrations of renin and aldosterone.

Further reading

Beale R. Weaning from mechanical ventilation. *Br J Intens Care* 1994; **4**:168–175.

Pang D, Keenan S, Cook DJ, Sibbald WJ. The effect of positive pressure airway support on mortality and the need for intubation in cardiogenic pulmonary edema: a systemic review. *Chest* 1998; **114**:1185–92.

Pinsky MR. Cardiovascular effects of ventilatory support and withdrawal. *Anaesth Analg* 1994; **79**:567–76.

Ranien VM, Eissna NT, Corbeil C *et al.* Effects of positive end-expiratory pressure on alveolar recruitment and gas exchange in patients with the adult respiratory distress syndrome. *Am Rev Respir Dis* 1991; **144**:544–51.

Tusman G, Boehm SH, Vazquez de Anda GF, do Campo JL, Lachmann B. Alveolar recruitment strategy improves arterial oxygenation during general anaesthesia. *Br J Anaesth* 1999; **82**:8–13.

13 Pulmonary oedema

Describe the causes and treatment of pulmonary oedema.

Pulmonary oedema is the extravascular accumulation of fluid within a lung. In health, the lymphatics return normal leakage of fluid from capillaries to the intravascular space. This mechanism can fail, resulting in accumulation of fluid in the interstitial tissues, and the fluid can overflow into the alveolar spaces.

The *Starling equation* is fundamental to understanding these fluid shifts across capillaries. It describes the balance between oncotic and hydrostatic pressures between the intravascular and extravascular spaces:

$$J_v = K_f(P_{mv} - P_i) - (TT_{mv} - T_{ti})$$

where

J_v = fluid flux out of the pulmonary capillary
K_f = filtration coefficient for pulmonary capillaries
P_{mv} = pulmonary microvascular pressure
P_i = pulmonary oncotic pressure
TT_{mv} = microvascular oncotic pressure
T_{ti} = reflection coefficient that describes the permeability of a membrane to a molecule.

Presentation

Pulmonary oedema presents as shortness of breath, orthopnoea, paroxysmal nocturnal dyspnoea and a cough productive of blood-tinged frothy fluid. Clinical findings typically are fine inspiratory crackles on auscultation of the chest. Gas exchange is impaired. Chest x-ray appearance may include:
- distended upper-lobe veins
- Kerley B septal lines which are short horizontal lines at the periphery of the lower zone
- Kerley A septal lines which are long fine lines in the upper zone radiating from the hilum
- diffuse hazy shadowing radiating from the hilar region, mostly above the fissure and in the lower zone ('bat's wing' distribution is characteristic)
- small pleural effusions
- cardiac enlargement.

Aetiology

Causes of pulmonary oedema are:

- raised pulmonary capillary pressure
- decreased oncotic pressure
- increased capillary permeability
- obstruction of lymphatic drainage
- rapid lung expansion
- neurogenic oedema
- re-establishment of pulmonary perfusion
- high altitude.

In the management of pulmonary oedema, the likely cause should be sought to aim therapy at the underlying physiological abnormality.

Raised pulmonary capillary pressure occurs with an increase in left-sided preload. This may be due to left ventricular failure or mitral stenosis. Thus P_{mv} increases and hence J_v will increase. With a decrease in oncotic pressure, P_i decreases and hence the Starling equation is pushed to the left. It occurs primarily with hypoalbuminaemia seen in liver disease, protein loss and severe catabolism.

Capillary permeability is increased in sepsis, disseminated intravascular coagulation (DIC), systemic inflammatory respiratory syndrome (SIRS), fat embolism, by drugs, or following insult to the lung such as pulmonary aspiration or following inhalation of toxins.

The lymphatic drainage returns the fluid flux out of the pulmonary capillary back to the intravascular space. Obstruction of the lymphatic system due to any cause can impair this return and lead to pulmonary oedema. Increased superior vena caval pressure may also impair the lymphatic return.

A negative pressure in the interstitial tissues due to rapid lung expansion can lead to development of pulmonary oedema. This is sometimes seen in children following the relief of upper airway obstruction. It may also occur following rapid drainage of a pneumothorax.

A large surge of sympathetic overactivity occasionally follows head injury, resulting in neurogenic pulmonary oedema. The exact mechanism is poorly understood, but it may be due to rapid alteration in haemodynamic pressures.

Exercise at high altitude can lead to hypoxic pulmonary vasoconstriction and pulmonary oedema.

14 Ventilatory support

> Outline the modes of ventilatory support available for a patient with compromised respiratory function.

There are two commonly used forms of ventilation to support patients with compromised respiratory function:
- non-invasive ventilation
- invasive ventilation requiring endotracheal intubation.

Non-invasive ventilation

Non-invasive positive-pressure ventilation (NIPPV) is a method of respiratory support that can be provided by standard ventilators via a facemask. Most clinical practice with NIPPV is in managing chronic stable respiratory failure, but experience is growing in its use in the management of acute disease. NIPPV is gaining a place as a therapeutic option for patients who would otherwise be intubated. The indications for NIPPV are:

1. It avoids intubation in acute hypercapnic respiratory failure.
2. It circumvents the need for tracheotomy in patients recovering from critical illness or surgery.
3. It improves the preoperative cardiorespiratory function in patients with chronic ventilatory failure.
4. It facilitates weaning from mechanical ventilation.
5. It acts as a 'bridge' to transplantation in patients with end-stage respiratory failure.

The use of NIPPV has been described in:
- chronic obstructive pulmonary disease (COPD)
- chest wall disorders
- pneumonia
- cardiac failure
- cystic fibrosis
- obstructive sleep apnoea
- asthma
- postoperative ventilatory support.

There are several potential advantages in avoiding the need for endotracheal intubation. Intubation requires general anaesthesia and neuromuscular blockade, and it is often associated with a period of uncontrolled haemodynamic instability. Endotracheal intubation often requires the patient to be sedated, necessitates nasogastric or even parenteral feeding, and limits patient mobility and communication. Despite this, there are patients for whom endotracheal intubation remains mandatory.

The incidence of weaning failure is up to 20% of ventilated patients. In a small group of patients weaning is a lengthy process when recovery from organ failure occurs leaving only weaning to be accomplished. NIPPV can de-escalate treatment and allow patients to spend time free from the ventilator.

Requirements for NIPPV
1. Normal bulbar function.
2. A patient able to breathe spontaneously for at least 5 minutes.
3. Minimal sputum production.
4. Low requirement for supplemental oxygen.
5. Stable haemodynamic status.
6. A functioning gastrointestinal tract.

Invasive ventilation

When NIPPV is not possible a patient with respiratory failure will require endotracheal intubation and intermittent positive-pressure ventilation (IPPV). The indications for endotracheal intubation are:
- impaired conscious level (Glasgow coma score <8)
- loss of bulbar reflexes
- significant risk of aspiration
- potential loss of upper-airway integrity (oedema, thermal injury etc.).

The principal difference between positive-pressure ventilation and spontaneous breathing is that an increased airway pressure forcing gas into the lungs replaces the normal subatmospheric pressure, which draws air in.

The physiological changes during IPPV which affect gas exchange are:
- increased spread of V/Q ratios
- increased venous admixture
- increased V_D to V_T ratio (deadspace:tidal volume)
- decreased functional residual capacity (FRC) with possible encroachment on closing volume and alteration of regional compliance distribution in lungs
- lack of cough and sigh function
- inhibition of secretion clearance resulting from ciliary dysfunction.

The practice of artificial ventilation

The practice of artificial ventilation (either invasive or non-invasive) has developed from the use of simple IPPV to include a range of new techniques. These include the use of:
- PEEP and continuous positive airway pressure (CPAP)
- mandatory ventilation
- inverse-ratio ventilation
- high-frequency ventilation.

PEEP

PEEP is the maintenance of a positive pressure within the lungs throughout expiration and this may be applied during IPPV or NIPPV. This is the most direct way of recruiting non-ventilated alveoli; it is titrated to maintain an adequate tissue oxygen delivery with an acceptable inspired oxygen concentration. Optimal values for PEEP and tidal volumes can be determined from static pressure/volume curves. The actions of PEEP that explain the improvement in oxygenation are:

- re-expansion of collapsed alveoli
- redistribution of fluid to the more compliant perivascular space
- layering of fluid within the alveoli.

When the recruited airways are continually splintered open, alveolar wall shear stresses are much reduced and alveoli are no longer collapsing during every expiration, reducing the degree of volume-related lung injury.

Mandatory ventilation techniques (IMV, SIMV, MMV)

These allow the patient to breathe spontaneously while the mechanical ventilator maintains a preset level of ventilation.

The principle of *intermittent mandatory ventilation* (IMV) is that the patient receives a preset number of breaths of known tidal volume (V_T) from the ventilator and can in addition breathe spontaneously.

Synchronised intermittent mandatory ventilation (SIMV) synchronises the mandatory breaths from the ventilator with those of the patient. The efficiency of the synchronisation depends on the sensitivity of the ventilator in detecting spontaneous breathing and the rapidity with which a machine breath can be initiated.

Mandatory minute-ventilation (MMV) allows the patient to breathe spontaneously and no mechanical support is given unless the minute-ventilation decreases below a preset level. In this event the ventilator maintains the preset minimum with appropriate numbers of preset tidal volumes. The patient may thus receive the MMV either spontaneously, as a combination of spontaneous and artificial ventilation, or completely artificially if spontaneous activity ceases.

Advantages of IMV, SIMV and MMV

1. *Lower mean airway pressures.*
2. *Reduced sedation requirements.*
3. Avoidance of respiratory alkalosis.
4. More uniform/physiological intrapulmonary gas distribution.
5. Easier weaning from mechanical ventilation.
6. Reduced respiratory muscle atrophy and incoordination.
7. Reduced risk of cardiac decompensation during weaning.

Disadvantages of IMV, SIMV and MMV

1. *Increased risk of respiratory acidosis if there is no response to increased ventilatory demands.*
2. Possible increase in the work of breathing dependent on the resistance to flow in the spontaneous respiration circuit.
3. Respiratory muscle fatigue.
4. Prolongation of weaning if IMV not decreased aggressively.

Inverse-ratio ventilation

The rationale behind the use of an extended inspiratory time is to manipulate the pattern of applied pressure to achieve lung recruitment without causing over-inflation of the relatively normal alveoli. The overall effect of inverse-ratio ventilation (IRV) in patients is rather unpredictable and therapy must be carefully individualised. The potential benefits are considerable.

Usually IRV is used only when it is impossible to achieve acceptable oxygenation with conventional ventilator parameters. Attempts to prolong the inspiratory time in these patients should be made gradually since these patients are already unstable and rapid institution of this ventilatory strategy can precipitate a crisis. Many of the benefits of IRV can be achieved by changing the I:E ratio to 1:1 rather than formally reversing the I:E ratio.

High-frequency ventilation

Conventional approaches to mechanical ventilation attempt to duplicate the normal bulk flow of gas, with tidal volumes and frequencies in or near the psychological range. As lung function deteriorates, conventional strategies frequently fail to provide adequate CO_2 clearance or O_2 delivery without considerable potential for barotrauma or cardiovascular depression.

High-frequency ventilation (HFV) comprises three ventilatory techniques depending on the ventilatory frequency used. HFV is characterised by the use of small tidal volumes – in some circumstances less than anatomical deadspace. As a consequence of the smaller tidal volumes, the peak airway pressures are lower than with conventional ventilation, although the product of frequency and tidal volume is far greater.

The arguments in favour of the use of HFV generally hinge around the reduction in pressure swings which may reduce the incidence of barotrauma, and the improvement in ventilation and perfusion matching consequent on the different gas-delivery technique.

Factors affecting the tidal volume of HFV are:

- jet driving pressure
- injector size
- inspiratory time
- frequency

- size of endotracheal tube
- presence of entrainment gas
- presence of auto PEEP.

Clearly, with jet ventilation, as T_V approaches or becomes less than V_D (dead-space) gas transport has to occur by a different method than in conventional ventilation. Methods of gas transport during jet ventilation could be:

- bulk flow
- pendelluft
- coaxial flow
- Taylor dispersal
- molecular diffusion.

Although the relative importance of these mechanisms is unclear, bulk flow still accounts for appreciable gas transport especially near to the major airways. Pendelluft gas may be particularly pronounced in lungs with marked heterogeneity. It is likely that the contributions of the different mechanisms will change according to differences in lung pathology and ventilator settings.

The major problems related to the use of jet ventilation are due to inadequate humidification, physical damage due to jet impingement, and gas trapping.

Further reading

Benhamou D, Girault C, Fauré C et al. Nasal mask ventilation in acute respiratory failure. *Chest* 1992; **102**:912–17.

Brochand L. Non-invasive ventilation: practice issues (editorial comment). *Intens Care Med* 1993; **19**:431–2.

Brochand L, Mancebo J, Wysocke M et al. Non-invasive ventilation for acute exacerbation of chronic obstructive pulmonary disease. *N Engl J Med* 1995; **333**:817–22.

Butler R, Keenan SP, Inman KJ, Sibbald WJ, Block G. Is there a preferred technique for weaning the difficult-to-wean patient? A systemic review of the literature. *Crit Care Med* 1999; **27**:2331–6.

Carlton GC, Howland WS, Ray C et al. High-frequency jet ventilation: a prospective randomised evaluation. *Chest* 1993; **84**:551–9.

Garfield MJ. Non-invasive ventilation. *BJA CEPD Rev* 2001; **1**:142–5.

Pinsky MR. Cardiovascular effects of ventilatory support and withdrawal. *Anaesth Analg* 1994; **79**:567–76.

Stewart TE, Meade MO, Cook DJ et al. Evaluation of a ventilation strategy to prevent barotraumas in patients at high risk for acute respiratory distress syndrome. *N Engl J Med* 1998; **338**:355–61.

15 Burns

> Outline the management within the first 24 hours of a patient who receives 60% burns in a house fire.

Tissue damage due to burns can be due to either direct thermal injury or secondary injury from inflammatory mediators. Management is supportive as well as directed at avoiding and treating secondary complications.

The airway

Mucosal damage from upper-airway burns can be fatal. Check for signs of upper-airway obstruction. There is a low threshold for endotracheal intubation as upper-airway oedema can lead to complete airway obstruction within 24 hours of thermal injury. Facial oedema developing later can make endotracheal intubation very difficult.

Indicators of upper-airway burn are voice changes, chest x-ray changes due to inhalation injury, carboxyhaemoglobinaemia >15% (carbon monoxide poisoning). Consider dexamethasone IV to reduce oedema.

Breathing

Burns can lead to reduced chest wall compliance, reduced pulmonary compliance and reduced FRC.

Carbon monoxide poisoning is common in house fires. Carbon monoxide has 250 times the affinity of oxygen for haemoglobin. Symptoms of CO poisoning are headache and malaise (%HbCO 10–20), nausea and vomiting (%HbCO 30–40) and CVS collapse and death (%HbCO >60–70). In severe cases hyperbaric oxygen therapy should be considered.

Cyanide poisoning can also be a consequence of a house fire because it is released by burning certain plastics. Cyanide poisoning gives rise to a metabolic acidosis and arterial hypoxaemia. Severe cases can be treated with dicobalt edetate, a cyanide chelating agent, or with sodium thiosulphate which accelerates cyanide metabolism.

Cardiovascular system

Substantial amounts of water, protein and sodium are lost within the first 48 hours due to capillary bed leakage. Increased capillary leakage leads to generalised tissue oedema. There is a risk of profound hypovolaemia and hypotension. Fluid loss is maximal in the first few hours and returns to basal levels by 36 hours. Later, hypermetabolic state may lead to increase in cardiac output. Hypertension may occur secondary to renin and catecholamine release.

Fluid replacement

Intravenous fluid resuscitation is started in adults with greater than 15% burns and in children with greater than 10% burns. The crystalloid/colloid argument continues in the fluid management of burns patients. There are three commonly used formulae:

- *Mount Vernon formula*
  - The dose is colloid 0.5 mL/kg per 1% of burn coverage, given at 4-hour intervals for the first 12 hours, then at 6-hour intervals for the next 12 hours.
- *Parkland formula*
  - The dose is crystalloid 4 mL/kg per 1% of burn coverage. Half is given over the first 8 hours, and the remaining two quarters in the next two 8-hour periods.
- *Brook formula*
  - The dose per 1% of burn coverage is colloid 0.5 mL/kg plus crystalloid 1.5 mL/kg. Half of this fluid volume is given over the first 8 hours, and the remaining two quarters over the next two 8-hour periods.

Note that these regimes are in addition to normal daily fluid requirements.

Electrolytes, haematocrit, urine and plasma osmolality are checked regularly. Blood is transfused if the haematocrit falls below 0.3 or if haemoglobin concentration falls below 8.0 g/dL.

Other considerations

Hypothermia

Heat lost through burns leads to a rapid onset of hypothermia. There is, furthermore, impaired homeostatic control as a result of burn injury. This can be accentuated by infusion of large volumes of cold fluid. Measures include keeping the room temperature above 30°C and using blood warmers and heating mattresses.

Infection

Patients are at high risk of infection owing to loss of the skin barrier and generalized immunosuppression. Topical antimicrobial prophylaxis with flamazine cream and meticulous infection control nursing routines can avoid cross-infection. Systemic antibiotics are not used routinely.

Nutrition

Nasogastric feeding may be necessary. A nasojejunal tube should be considered if gastric stasis is present. A calorie to nitrogen ratio of 100:1 is commonly used. A hypercatabolic state requires early feeding.

Analgesia

Give as much intravenous opiate as necessary to keep the patient comfortable.

Full-thickness burns

Early debridement is advocated to avoid wound colonization and septic shock. However, extensive debridement may result in a large loss of blood.

Multiple-choice questions: The ICU

1. Total parenteral nutrition for an average adult should include:
   a) magnesium
   b) 14 grams of nitrogen daily
   c) 1 mL water for each kcal
   d) fat solutions in hepatic failure
   e) glucose.
2. In carbon monoxide poisoning the following are seen:
   a) arrhythmias
   b) hypotension
   c) extensor plantars
   d) cyanosis
   e) hyperventilation.
3. Pulmonary oxygen toxicity during oxygen therapy is associated with:
   a) prolonged exposure
   b) high altitude
   c) increased muscle activity
   d) increased carbon dioxide tension
   e) anaemia.
4. Oxygen toxicity to the lung is due to:
   a) inspired oxygen (F_1O_2) above 0.6
   b) prolonged exposure
   c) increased arterial partial pressure of oxygen
   d) the effect of oxygen on pulmonary vessels
   e) unhumidified oxygen.
5. At 30°C:
   a) Oxygen consumption is one-third that at 37°C
   b) Oxygen solubility is raised
   c) J-waves might appear on the ECG
   d) Active rewarming should be commenced
   e) Carbon dioxide solubility is reduced.
6. A thyrotoxic crisis should be immediately treated by:
   a) Radioactive iodine
   b) Propranolol
   c) Diazepam
   d) Lugol's iodine
   e) Adrenaline.

7. Appropriate management of an acute head injury includes:
   a) Naloxone
   b) Methylprednisolone 30 mg/kg
   c) Hyperventilation to a P_aCO_2 of 3.3–4 kPa
   d) Mannitol 2 mg/kg
   e) Burr holes.
8. Helium:
   a) is useful in treating bronchospasm
   b) is stored as liquid in brown cylinders
   c) has a lower viscosity than oxygen
   d) causes an alteration in voice
   e) supports combustion.
9. A poor prognosis in tetanus is associated with:
   a) a long incubation period
   b) minimal muscle damage
   c) distal injury
   d) severe muscle spasm
   e) previous immunisation.
10. In patients with haemorrhagic shock:
    a) physiological dead-space is increased
    b) renal blood flow is decreased
    c) antidiuretic hormone (ADH) secretion is increased
    d) the oxygen dissociation curve is shifted to the left
    e) oxygen delivery is decreased.
11. Recognised effects of PEEP include:
    a) sodium retention
    b) fall in cardiac output
    c) rise in closing volume
    d) rise in FRC
    e) fall in CVP.
12. Raised left ventricular end-diastolic pressure (LVEDP) implies:
    a) increased left ventricular compliance
    b) decreased left ventricular systemic work index (LVSWI)
    c) decreased oxygen flux
    d) decreased myocardial oxygen demand
    e) decreased myocardial oxygen supply.
13. Pulmonary capillary wedge pressure (PCWP) is a reliable parameter:
    a) in mitral stenosis
    b) after anterior myocardial infarction
    c) in pulmonary stenosis
    d) in aortic stenosis
    e) in pulmonary fibrosis.

14. In septic shock:
    a) peripheral hypothermia is associated with a good prognosis
    b) the patients usually have an increased cardiac output
    c) the patients usually have a depleted circulating volume
    d) the causative organisms are always Gram-negative
    e) antibiotics should not be given before blood culture results are available.

15. An 8-year-old child is rescued 20 minutes after drowning and has a core temperature of 30°C and fixed dilated pupils. Further appropriate treatment includes:
    a) phenobarbitone
    b) rapid rewarming
    c) hypoventilation
    d) steroids
    e) cardiopulmonary resuscitation.

16. The following findings occur with a large pulmonary embolus:
    a) an increase in pulmonary artery pressure
    b) an increase in right ventricular pressure
    c) an increase in left atrial pressure
    d) an increase in physiological dead-space
    e) a decrease in right atrial pressure.

17. Increased left ventricular end-diastolic pressure:
    a) causes increased compliance of the left ventricle
    b) causes decreased tension in left ventricular wall
    c) causes decreased left ventricular stroke work index
    d) occurs in mitral stenosis
    e) is associated with raised pulmonary artery pressure.

18. In the oxygen dissociation curve, causes of a right shift include:
    a) low-molecular-weight dextran
    b) digitalis
    c) metabolic acidosis
    d) respiratory alkalosis
    e) hypoxia.

19. An increased alveolar–arterial (A–a) gradient is associated with:
    a) an increased F_iO_2
    b) a decreased F_iO_2
    c) a decreased FRC
    d) an increased V/Q ratio
    e) an increased shunt.

20. Complications of PEEP include:
   a) alteration of the alveolar–arterial (A–a) gradient
   b) decreased cardiac output
   c) increased renal output
   d) pneumothorax in an emphysematous patient
   e) hypercarbia.

21. PEEP added to intermittent mandatory ventilation (IMV) is indicated:
   a) to hasten weaning
   b) if it has already been used for IPPV
   c) if $F_IO_2 > 0.6$ and $P_aO_2 < 10\,kPa$
   d) if respiratory rate is greater than 30 breaths per minute
   e) if PCWP $> 8\,mmHg$.

22. PEEP:
   a) decreases cardiac output
   b) increases CVP
   c) increases closing volume
   d) increases FRC
   e) decreases P_vO_2.

23. Pulmonary artery capillary wedge pressure can be increased:
   a) after myocardial infarction
   b) in mitral stenosis
   c) in aortic regurgitation
   d) in pulmonary fibrosis
   e) in pulmonary stenosis.

24. In early sepsis syndrome:
   a) cardiac output is normal
   b) a decreased white cell count is a poor prognostic sign
   c) ACTH levels are low
   d) insulin is raised
   e) P_aO_2 is lowered.

25. Features of dissemated intravascular coagulation include:
   a) a lowered fibrinogen level
   b) a normal prothrombin time and activated partial thromboplastin time
   c) heparin a reasonable treatment following placental abruption
   d) may occur secondary to malaria
   e) may have a compensated phase with no bleeding.

26. Gram-negative septicaemic shock is associated with:
   a) urine output $< 0.5\,mL/kg$ per hour
   b) disseminated intravascular coagulation
   c) hypotension unresponsive to fluid loading
   d) high fever
   e) diminished cardiac output.

27. An increased alveolar–arterial (A–a) oxygen difference is caused by:
    a) a decreased FRC
    b) increased inspired oxygen
    c) nitrous oxide absorption
    d) hepatic failure
    e) increased V–Q mismatch.

28. Essential criteria for the diagnosis of brainstem death are:
    a) equal pupils
    b) absent doll's head response
    c) absent limb movements
    d) patient's temperature must exceed 35°C
    e) P_aCO_2 must exceed 6.5 kPa at completion of apnoea testing.

29. An adult breathing 100% oxygen at sea level may suffer from:
    a) retrosternal chest pain
    b) convulsions
    c) dizziness
    d) atelectasis
    e) permanent visual damage.

Answers to multiple-choice questions

	a)	b)	c)	d)	e)
1.	a) True;	b) True;	c) True;	d) True;	e) True
2.	a) True;	b) True;	c) True;	d) False;	e) True
3.	a) True;	b) False;	c) False;	d) False;	e) False
4.	a) True;	b) True;	c) False;	d) True;	e) False
5.	a) False;	b) True;	c) True;	d) False;	e) False
6.	a) False;	b) True;	c) True;	d) False;	e) False
7.	a) False;	b) False;	c) True;	d) False;	e) True
8.	a) False;	b) True;	c) True;	d) True;	e) False
9.	a) False;	b) False;	c) False;	d) True;	e) True
10.	a) True;	b) True;	c) True;	d) False;	e) True
11.	a) True;	b) True;	c) False;	d) True;	e) False
12.	a) False;	b) False;	c) True;	d) False;	e) True
13.	a) False;	b) True;	c) True;	d) True;	e) False
14.	a) False;	b) True;	c) True;	d) False;	e) False
15.	a) False;	b) True;	c) False;	d) False;	e) True
16.	a) True;	b) True;	c) False;	d) True;	e) False
17.	a) False;	b) False;	c) False;	d) False;	e) False
18.	a) False;	b) False;	c) True;	d) False;	e) True
19.	a) True;	b) False;	c) True;	d) True;	e) True
20.	a) True;	b) True;	c) False;	d) True;	e) False
21.	a) True;	b) True;	c) True;	d) False;	e) False
22.	a) True;	b) True;	c) False;	d) True;	e) False
23.	a) True;	b) True;	c) True;	d) False;	e) False
24.	a) True;	b) True;	c) False;	d) True;	e) True
25.	a) True;	b) False;	c) False;	d) True;	e) True
26.	a) True;	b) True;	c) True;	d) False;	e) True
27.	a) True;	b) True;	c) True;	d) True;	e) True
28.	a) False;	b) True;	c) False;	d) True;	e) True
29.	a) True;	b) False;	c) False;	d) True;	e) False

NEUROANAESTHESIA

1   Head injury

> Describe the initial hospital treatment of a 40-year-old man with an acute head injury.

Head injuries account for the majority of deaths from trauma in the UK. It is estimated that of the 165 000 new cases per year in the UK, approximately 15 000 are classified as severe to moderately severe. Of these patients, 7.5% die while 20% survive with significant residual disability. Road traffic accidents account for more than 50% of severe head injuries, and cause 70% of deaths.

Brain injury is either primary or secondary. Primary injury occurs at the time of the initial trauma and is usually considered to be irreversible, whereas secondary injury occurs after the time of initial trauma. Much of the anaesthetic management of severely head-injured patients is aimed at preventing or reducing secondary brain injury.

Causes of secondary brain injury are:

- *Intracranial*
    - elevated intracranial pressure (ICP)
    - convulsions
    - pyrexia
    - biochemical events such as free radical formation.
- *Systemic*
    - depressed arterial pressure
    - depressed arterial O_2 tension.

The prevention of secondary brain injury is dependent upon adequate oxygen delivery to the endangered tissue. The key to anaesthetic management is thus avoidance of systemic hypoxia and hypertension.

Fifteen per cent of patients with severe head injury have cervical spinal cord injury. Incautious manipulation of the head and neck in these patients may lead to permanent and disabling damage to the cervical spinal cord. A normal lateral cervical spine x-ray does not exclude spinal injury. The neck is protected with a hard cervical collar, sandbags are placed each side of the head and neck, and the forehead is firmly taped to each side of the bed or trolley.

Neurological disability should be assessed only when the airway, breathing and circulation (ABC) have been assessed and secured. The purpose of neurological assessment in the primary survey is to determine the severity and type of injury. This will determine immediate management. Neurological consultation should not be delayed by diagnostic examinations such as computed tomography (CT) scanning. The Glasgow Coma Score (GCS) should be used to quantify conscious level in all severely injured patients. Severe head injury is often defined as a GCS of 8 or less.

Injuries of force sufficient to damage the intracranial contents may often be associated with seemingly unconnected injuries of the abdomen, chest or pelvis. Unconscious patients are at risk of aspiration of gastric contents.

The severely head-injured patient often requires tracheal intubation and mechanical ventilation (see under INDICATIONS FOR REFERRAL OF HEAD INJURY, page 174). Neurological assessment such as localising (lateralising) signs should be recorded before administering anaesthesia. Nasal intubation should not be attempted because of the risk of unrecognised injury to the cribriform plate. The simplest method of securing the airway is with an oral endotracheal tube placed via direct visualisation of the larynx. In the patient with severe facial injuries, a cricothyroidotomy may be required. A rapid-sequence induction with properly applied cricoid pressure is the preferred method, as most patients will be at significant risk of regurgitation of gastric contents. An assistant should provide in-line manual stabilisation of the neck by firmly grasping both sides of the patient's head and keeping it motionless during the procedure.

Induction technique

Following pre-oxygenation, any induction agent may be used except ketamine, which produces a rise in ICP. Significant hypertension on induction should be avoided. Suxamethonium is commonly used to provide muscle relaxation despite its tendency to increase ICP. A short-acting opioid such as alfentanil will blunt the potentially damaging arterial and intracranial hypertensive response to laryngoscopy.

Once intubated, the patient's lungs should be mechanically ventilated. An orogastric tube should be passed and the stomach emptied. Muscle relaxation is used to prevent coughing and massive surges in ICP. The delivered inspired oxygen concentration should be as high as is required to provide a normal arterial oxygen saturation. Positive end-expiratory pressure (PEEP) increases intrathoracic pressure and may impede jugular venous drainage. If it is required it should be kept to a minimum.

Additional injuries must be sought and circulatory blood volume restored as quickly as possible. It is extremely rare for a cranial injury to be the sole cause of hypotension. Fluid resuscitation is accomplished with saline 0.9%, colloid and cross-matched blood. There may be severe lability in the cardiovascular system owing to the large surges of catecholamines seen after head injury.

The bed should be tilted into a 20-degree reverse Trendelenburg position and any constriction, including tracheal tubes, should be removed from around the neck. Elevated ICP may be effectively controlled by pharmacological means. Mannitol (0.25–1 g/kg) is frequently used for this purpose. Steroids have no role in the acutely head injured patient.

The patient's oxygen delivery must be kept as near normal as possible, by maintaining the cardiac output and keeping $P_aO_2 > 13$ kPa and haemoglobin >120 g/L. Cerebral perfusion pressure (CPP) should be kept as close to 70 mmHg as possible. When CPP is critical, ICP can be monitored directly by insertion of either an intraventricular line (most accurate, but most invasive), a subdural catheter or a hollow bolt. Doppler measurement of cerebral blood flow and jugular bulb oximetry are currently under evaluation as monitoring techniques. Both give information regarding the adequacy of cerebral blood flow and may result in a more rational, goal-directed approach to management.

Inotropes and vasoconstrictors may be useful in elevating arterial pressure and hence CPP. Noradrenaline is commonly used in this context. Care must be taken to avoid renal hypoperfusion. Additionally, there is a concern that injured areas of the brain may allow the passage of noradrenaline via a leaky blood–brain barrier and suffer damaging local vasoconstriction.

Mechanical hyperventilation is useful in acutely lowering ICP. The duration of its effect is approximately 4–8 hours since the cerebrospinal fluid pH is actively restored by the retention of protons. Little benefit is gained below a P_aCO_2 of 3.5 kPa. Because of the danger of vasoconstriction leading to cerebral ischaemia, its use should be restricted to moderate hyperventilation to a P_aCO_2 of 3.5–4.5 kPa.

The cerebral metabolic rate for oxygen ($CMRO_2$) may exceed cerebral oxygen supply. The head-injured patient is prone to epileptiform convulsions. These dramatically increase $CMRO_2$ and must be prevented. Phenytoin infusions are often used as prophylaxis with a slow loading dose of 15 mg/kg. Acutely, seizures must be terminated as quickly as possible and thiopentone and diazepam are effective. Etomidate provides a good balance of cardiovascular stability and anticonvulsant properties. Core temperature should be monitored and pyrexia controlled urgently. The blood glucose should be maintained at between 5–15 mmol/L as hypoglycaemia and hyperglycaemia may reduce survival from severe traumatic brain injury.

Other measures aimed at cerebral protection currently under evaluation include the use of pharmacological agents (N-methyl-D-aspartate), receptor antagonists, free radical scavengers, calcium-channel blockers and therapeutic hypothermia.

2 Intracranial pressure (ICP) measurement

> **Discuss the measurement of intracranial pressure and the techniques available for reducing it.**

There are three primary reasons for monitoring the injured brain in the intensive care unit (ICU):
* to detect harmful pathophysiological events before they cause irreversible damage to the brain
* to diagnose and treat the harmful pathophysiological event
* to provide feedback to guide therapy.

Intracranial pressure (ICP) is often monitored in specialised neuro intensive care units. It was first introduced into clinical practice about 30 years ago and has been most widely used as an adjunct to the treatment of severely head-injured patients. Almost all neurotrauma patients who die demonstrate ischaemic damage at post-mortem, much of which is generally believed to be secondary and occurring after initial injury.

ICP rises when the compensatory mechanisms, which control ICP within the rigid skull vault, are overcome. In acute brain injury compliance is lost, so that a small change in cerebral volume may lead to a rapid rise in ICP, thereby reducing cerebral perfusion pressure (CPP) with a consequent risk of secondary ischaemic brain injury.

After a head injury or subarachnoid haemorrhage, ICP commonly rises up to 20 mmHg even when computed tomography (CT) appearances are normal. In health, ICP varies between 5 and 10 mmHg in the supine position.

Intervention is required if pressures rise to greater than 20 mmHg for more than 10–20 minutes.

ICP monitoring

Two methods of ICP monitoring are commonly employed in clinical practice:
* fluid-filled catheters
* transducer-tipped systems.

Intraventricular fluid-filled catheters allow direct measurement of ICP and have the added advantage of allowing CSF (cerebrospinal fluid) withdrawal when ICP rises. Placement may be difficult in the lateral ventricles when the ventricle is small, as is usual after trauma. Subdural catheters have their advocates and may be easily inserted after craniotomy to allow direct postoperative ICP monitoring. The disadvantages of this technique are of damping by the swollen brain, signal drift, limited frequency response and a tendency to blockage, thus presenting an infection risk. Extradural probes have not been widely adopted, as there is uncertainty about the relationship between ICP and pressure in the extradural space.

Transducer-tipped systems, although more costly, have the advantage of measuring CSF or intra-parenchymal pressures with high accuracy, minimal drift over a long period and good frequency response. The microtransducer is secured through a support bolt inserted via a twist-drill hole in the skull, and sealed with an airtight seal. Some systems can be tunnelled subcutaneously. Additional information can be acquired by analysis of the ICP waveform allowing deductions about craniospherical compliance. The ICP pulse wave is generated by the arterial blood pressure. Slow decay in the diastolic component is an indicator of a tight, stiff non-compliant brain, whereas the slack compliant healthy brain will demonstrate a sinusoidal diastolic slope.

Techniques for reducing ICP

The following are methods in use:
- reverse Trendelenberg position
- removal of any constriction around the neck
- mannitol
- positive-pressure ventilation
- blood pressure control
- frusemide
- removal of any space-occupying lesion.

The cranium is, essentially, a rigid box containing the brain, the meninges, the cerebrospinal fluid and blood vessels. Any increase in the volume of any of its components will cause the intracranial pressure to rise. This relationship is known as the Monroe–Kelly hypothesis.

Cerebral blood flow is kept constant through a range of mean arterial pressures (MAP). This vascular autoregulation may be lost in traumatic brain injury. Cerebral blood flow is closely coupled to the cerebral metabolic requirement for oxygen ($CMRO_2$), supplies being adjusted to demand. Cerebral perfusion pressure (CPP) is defined as:

$$CPP = MAP - ICP.$$

Basic techniques may be effective in reducing the head-injured patient's elevated ICP. The bed should be tilted into a 20-degree reverse Trendelenberg position. The head should be kept in a neutral position and any constriction, including tracheal tube ties, should be removed from around the neck.

Elevated ICP may be treated with mannitol (0.25–1 g/kg). Its action is poorly understood, but probably consists of an osmotic effect, drawing water from the brain, and an effect in reducing blood viscosity, reducing intracranial blood volume for a given blood flow. Prolonged administration of mannitol may eventually lead to an increase in brain swelling, possibly due to leakage of mannitol across the blood–brain barrier.

Mechanical ventilation via an oral endotracheal tube is facilitated by muscle relaxation. Coughing, causing surges in ICP, or accidental extubation can thus be avoided. Minute-volume should be adjusted to keep a low-to-normal P_aCO_2 or $ETCO_2$ leading to cerebral vasoconstriction and reduction in intracranial blood volume and hence ICP. Vasoregulation is commonly dysfunctional in damaged areas of the brain, so flow tends to be maintained in these areas despite the lowered P_aCO_2. Mechanical hyperventilation is useful in acutely lowering ICP. The duration of its effect is approximately 4–8 hours since the CSF pH is actively restored by the retention of protons. Subsequent intracranial hypertension may be managed with further hyperventilation, but little benefit is gained below a P_aCO_2 of 3.5 kPa. Because of the danger of vasoconstriction leading to cerebral ischaemia, its use should be restricted to moderate hyperventilation, to a P_aCO_2 of 3.5–4.5 kPa unless additional monitoring is used (e.g. jugular bulb oximetry).

Severe lability in the cardiovascular system is sometimes seen following head injury, owing to surges of catecholamines. These should be treated pharmacologically to avoid surges in ICP. Excessive intravascular pressures may exacerbate vasogenic cerebral oedema. Hypertension can be just as damaging, however, as prevention of secondary brain injury is dependent upon adequate oxygen delivery to the endangered tissue.

Frusemide may be effective, but it is given as a second-line drug or in combination with mannitol since they appear to exhibit some synergism. It is now generally agreed that steroids have little role in the acute head-injured patient.

Removal of any pathological space-occupying lesion (such as haematoma) may be the definitive measure to reduce ICP.

Further reading

Clifton GL, Robertson CS, Kyper K et al. Cardiovascular response to severe head injury. J Neurosurg 1983; **59**:447–54.

Czosnyka M, Czosnyka Z, Pickard JD. Laboratory testing of three intracranial pressure mecrotransducers. Neurosurgery 1996; **38**:219–24.

Gaab MR, Heissler HE, Ehrahardt K. Physical characteristics of various methods of measuring ICP. In: Hoff JT, Betz ANL (eds), Intracranial Pressure, vol. 8. Berlin: Springer Verlag, 1989, pp. 16–21.

Ghajar J. Intracranial pressure monitoring techniques. New Horizons 1995; **3**:395–9.

Miller JD. Head injury and brain ischaemia: implications for therapy. Br J Anaesth 1985; **57**:120–30.

Wilkinson HA, Rosenfeld SR. Frusemide and mannitol in the treatment of acute experimental intracramial hypertension. Neurosurgery 1983; **12**: 405–10.

3 Indications for referral of head injury

List (a) the indications for intubation and ventilation of a head-injured patient, (b) indications for brain scan in a general hospital, and (c) what the neurosurgical centre needs to know about the head-injured patient you are referring.

Indications for intubation and ventilation

Intubation
1. To obtain a secure, clear airway.
2. To prevent aspiration of blood or gastric contents.
3. To facilitate mechanical ventilation.

Ventilation
1. $P_aO_2 < 10\,kPa$ with $F_IO_2 = 0.6$.
2. Hypoventilation ($P_aCO_2 > 5.5\,kPa$).
3. Spontaneous hyperventilation ($P_aO_2 < 3.0\,kPa$).
4. If sedation is required to tolerate the tracheal tube.
5. Uncontrolled convulsions.
6. Deteriorating neurological condition.
7. Glasgow Coma Score < 9.
8. Intracranial pressure >25 mmHg.
9. To allow adequate analgesia in the presence of multiple injuries.
10. To allow safe transport.

Indications for scanning in a general hospital

1. Confusion (GCS < 14) persisting after the initial assessment and resuscitation.
2. Unstable systemic state precluding transfer to neurosurgical centre.
3. Diagnosis uncertain.
4. Patient fully conscious but with a skull fracture, or following first fit (admit and consider head scan).

Criteria for neurosurgical referral of head-injured patients

Without preliminary head CT or MRI
1. Coma (not obeying commands) even after resuscitation, even without a skull fracture.
2. Deterioration in the level of consciousness of more than two GCS points, or progressive neurological deficit.
3. Open injury, depressed skull fracture, penetrating injury or basal skull fracture.

4. Tense fontanel in a child.
5. Patient fulfils criteria for scan, but this cannot be performed in a reasonable time (3–4 hours).

After brain scan in a general hospital
1. Abnormal scan (preferably after neurosurgical opinion on electronically transferred images).
2. Scan normal, but patient's progress unsatisfactory.

What the neurosurgical centre needs to know at referral

1. Patient's age and past medical history if known.
2. History of injury:
    Time of injury
    Cause and mechanism.
3. Neurological state:
    Talking or not after injury
    Consciousness level on arrival at A&E
    Trends in consciousness level after arrival.
4. Sequential GCS: pupil and limb response.
5. Cardiorespiratory state:
    Blood pressure and pulse rate
    Arterial blood gases, respiratory rate and pattern.
6. Injuries:
    Skull fracture
    Extracranial injuries.
7. Imaging findings: haematoma, swelling, other.
8. Management:
    Airway protection, ventilatory status
    Circulatory status and fluid therapy (mannitol)
    Treatment of associated injuries (?surgery)
    Monitoring
    Drug doses and times of administration.

Further reading
Gentleman D, Dearden M, Midgley S, Maclean D. Guidelines for resuscitation and transfer of patients with serious head injuries. *Br Med J* 1993; **307**:547–52.
Heiden JS, Weiss MH, Rosenberg AW *et al.* Management of cervical spinal cord trauma in Southern California. *J Neurosurg* 1975; **43**:732–6.
Jennett B. Assessment of the severity of head injury. *J Neurol Neurosurg Psychiatry* 1976; **39**:647–55.

Miller JD. Head injury and brain ischaemia: implications for therapy. *Br J Anaesth* 1985; **57**:120–30.

Rose J, Valtonen S, Jennett B. Avoidable factors contributing to death after head injury. *Br Med J* 1977; **ii**:615–18.

Teasdale G, Jennett B. Assessment of coma and impaired consciousness: a practical scale. *Lancet* 1974; **ii**:81–4.

4 Spinal cord injury

> What particular problems may occur during lower abdominal surgery in a patient who suffered a traumatic transection of the spinal cord at C6 four weeks previously? Briefly indicate how you would avoid or prevent the problems you describe.

Problems following cord transection at C6

These include:

- airway
- respiration
- cardiovascular
- abdominal
- biochemical
- temperature regulation
- infection
- pain management
- suxamethonium
- psychological difficulties.

Discussion

About 40% of paraplegic patients about to undergo surgery will require general anaesthesia, as it is difficult to be sure that the lesion of the cord is complete.

With a spinal cord transection at C6, patients may have impaired upper-airway protective reflexes with poor clearance of secretions. Vital capacity, respiratory muscle power and arterial oxygenation are decreased whilst residual volume and P_aCO_2 are increased. Respiratory complications such as broncho-pneumonia, pulmonary oedema and pulmonary embolism may occur. Phrenic nerve function will be preserved in this patient, and hence diaphragmatic function, as the origin of the phrenic nerve comes from C3 to C5.

C6 cord transection results in total sympathectomy whilst the parasympathetic system via the vagus nerve remains intact. This may result in hypertension, bradycardia and arrhythmias in the acute phase. Life-threatening autonomic hyperreflexia with uncontrolled sympathetic discharge may result in severe hypertension. Impaired vasoconstriction increases the susceptibility to postural hypertension and the haemodynamic effects of intermittent positive-pressure ventilation (IPPV). Ganglion blocking agents such as antagonists or direct vasodilators may be used for the control of blood pressure. Preload must be carefully monitored with central venous pressure or pulmonary capillary wedge pressure (PCWP) measurement.

Gastric stasis results in an increased risk of regurgitation and aspiration. Stress ulcers are common. Bladder atony results in permanent catheterisation with the considerable risk of urinary tract infection. Bowel atony may result in the need for manual faecal evacuation.

Decubitus ulceration and infection are common complications in quadraplegic patients. In the chronically injured state (after 4–8 weeks), muscle spasms and contractions may develop. Sympathectomy results in an inability to vasoconstrict and hypothermia can occur. Thus patients should be positioned carefully on the operating table both to protect pressure areas and to avoid excessive heat loss by taking necessary precautions.

Osteoporosis and hypercalcaemia occur in the chronic stage of injury. After 4 days, suxamethonium may cause life-threatening hyperkalaemia due to skeletal muscle denervation. The exact time when the risk of this complication disappears is uncertain. Suxamethonium should probably be avoided until 1 year after the injury. Hypoventilation due to inadequate respiratory function may result in respiratory acidosis, whilst fluid loss from the stomach can cause a metabolic hypokalaemic alkalosis.

These patients are often young and the psychological trauma of such an injury must be fully appreciated. In a patient with a 4-week-old C6 transection, the stability of the fracture site and possible complications of the injury must be assessed, particularly if intubation is planned. Pain management in these patients can be difficult. There may be some residual cord function involving pain pathways. Contractures and spasm may be very painful and patients often develop neuropathic pain.

Regional anaesthetic techniques decrease the incidence of autonomic hyperreflexic crisis. To prevent intraoperative spinal reflexes, muscle relaxants and IPPV are often required. A regional technique alone is not adequate for lower abdominal surgery. Cricoid pressure should always be used when intubating these patients owing to the high risk of regurgitation and aspiration.

Postoperative ventilation and cardiovascular support may be necessary to optimise respiratory function prior to extubation. Neuromuscular blocking drugs should be completely reversed prior to extubation since cough strength may be poor and secretions copious.

Further reading

Fraser A, Edmonds-Seal J. Spinal cord injuries. *Anaesthesia* 1982; **37**:1084–98.

Heath KJ. The effect on laryngoscopy of different cervical spine immobilisation techniques. *Anaesthesia* 1994; **49**:843–5.

Schonwald G *et al*. Cardiovascular complications during anaesthesia in chronic spinal cord injured patients. *Anaesthesiology* 1981; **55**:550–8.

Multiple-choice questions: Neuroanaesthesia

1. After head injury, increased intracranial pressure (ICP) is indicated by:
    a) a fall in systemic blood pressure
    b) a reduction of the Glasgow coma score
    c) an increase in heart rate
    d) an increase in P_aCO_2
    e) small pupils.

2. In the diagnosis of brainstem death:
    a) lack of EEG activity is essential
    b) caloric tests must be performed bilaterally
    c) the admitting consultant must certify death
    d) lack of stretch reflexes in all limbs is essential
    e) the pupils must be fixed and dilated.

3. A patient with a head injury becomes unconscious and develops signs of raised ICP. Management in the acute phase includes:
    a) craniotomy
    b) treatment with mannitol
    c) obtaining an electroencephalogram
    d) performing an immediate lumbar puncture
    e) ordering a digital subtraction angiogram.

4. The management of air embolism during posterior fossa surgery may include:
    a) positioning the patient on the right side
    b) administration of mannitol
    c) raising cerebral venous pressure
    d) discontinuation of nitrous oxide
    e) rapid infusion of fluid.

5. Regional cerebral metabolism is increased by
    a) halothane
    b) mannitol
    c) pain
    d) ketamine
    e) sodium thiopentone.

6. In the diagnosis of brainstem death:
    a) consultation with a neurologist is needed
    b) an EEG must be flat for 24 hours
    c) convulsions pre-empt the diagnosis
    d) spinal reflexes may be present
    e) blood must be sent for drug screening.

7. The following statements are true:
   a) CSF should be examined if a brain tumour is suspected
   b) CSF is characteristically normal in trigeminal neuralgia
   c) CSF protein greater than 1.5 g may be found in motor neurone disease
   d) CSF protein is raised in untreated meningococcal meningitis
   e) CSF cell count is increased in Guillain–Barré syndrome
8. Diplopia may occur in:
   a) myasthenia gravis
   b) retrobulbar neuritis
   c) cerebellar hemisphere disease
   d) Horner's syndrome
   e) multiple sclerosis.
9. In L5–S1 disc prolapse with sciatica in the right leg:
   a) loss of the knee jerk occurs on the right
   b) loss of sensation in the medial right calf occurs
   c) incontinence requires further surgical investigation
   d) plaster of paris cast is the preferred early treatment
   e) scoliosis is commonly associated.
10. Suitable anaesthetic techniques for patients with raised intracranial pressure are:
   a) nitrous oxide, oxygen and fentanyl; controlled ventilation
   b) nitrous oxide, oxygen, thiopentone and atracurium
   c) ketamine
   d) halothane, nitrous oxide and oxygen; spontaneous ventilation
   e) premedication with morphine.
11. Following a head injury, signs which suggest the need for urgent craniotomy include:
   a) reduced conscious level
   b) dilated pupil
   c) hypotension
   d) convulsions
   e) CSF rhinorrhoea.
12. A patient with paraplegia of recent onset with injury at T4 may have:
   a) hypotension on IPPV
   b) adductor spasm
   c) bradycardia
   d) hypothermia
   e) urinary retention.

13. The following are reliable indications of air embolism:
    a) a change in respiratory rate
    b) arryhthmias
    c) hypertension
    d) delta waves on EEG
    e) a mill wheel murmur.
14. In the early detection of air embolus, the following are useful:
    a) ECG
    b) ultrasound
    c) end-tidal CO_2
    d) fall in blood pressure
    e) change in ventilatory pattern.
15. The following may contribute to the development of a postoperative cauda equina syndrome:
    a) age
    b) the use of adrenalin in epidurals
    c) Trendelenberg position
    d) spinal barbotage
    e) marked intraoperative haemodilution.
16. Immediately after complete transection of the spinal cord, the following occur:
    a) flaccid paralysis with loss of sensation and reflexes
    b) loss of motor function and sensation with no loss of reflexes
    c) spasticity and increased reflexes
    d) loss of sensation but no loss of power
    e) loss of power but no loss of sensation.
17. Neuropraxia:
    a) is more common after long operations
    b) does not occur with local anaesthetics
    c) does not occur with muscle relaxants
    d) only occurs when previous neuropathy is present
    e) takes years to recover from.
18. In patients with increased ICP requiring a general anaesthetic, the following are especially dangerous:
    a) fentanyl, nitrous oxide/oxygen and controlled ventilation
    b) ketamine
    c) spontaneous ventilation with nitrous oxide/oxygen and halothane
    d) thiopentone/atracurium/ nitrous oxide/oxygen
    e) a total intravenous technique using propofol and remifentanil.

19. In a patient with a T4 injury, a safe technique for cystoscopy includes:
    a) no anaesthesia
    b) topical urethral local anaesthetic
    c) spinal anaesthesia
    d) thiopentone induction followed by nitrous oxide/oxygen/isoflurane anaesthesia
    e) a total intravenous technique using propofol and remifentanil.

Answers to multiple-choice questions

1.	a) False;	b) True;	c) False;	d) True;	e) False
2.	a) False;	b) False;	c) False;	d) False;	e) False
3.	a) True;	b) True;	c) False;	d) False;	e) False
4.	a) False;	b) False;	c) True;	d) True;	e) True
5.	a) False;	b) False;	c) True;	d) False;	e) False
6.	a) False;	b) False;	c) False;	d) True;	e) False
7.	a) False;	b) True;	c) False;	d) True;	e) False
8.	a) True;	b) False;	c) False;	d) False;	e) True
9.	a) False;	b) False;	c) True;	d) False;	e) False
10.	a) True;	b) True;	c) False;	d) False;	e) False
11.	a) False;	b) True;	c) False;	d) False;	e) False
12.	a) True;	b) False;	c) True;	d) True;	e) True
13.	a) True;	b) True;	c) False;	d) False;	e) False
14.	a) True;	b) True;	c) True;	d) False;	e) False
15.	a) True;	b) True;	c) False;	d) False;	e) True
16.	a) True;	b) False;	c) False;	d) False;	e) False
17.	a) True;	b) False;	c) False;	d) False;	e) False
18.	a) False;	b) True;	c) True;	d) False;	e) True
19.	a) False;	b) False;	c) True;	d) True;	e) True

Answers to multiple-choice questions

SECTION SIX

OBSTETRICS

1   Caesarean section in pre-eclampsia

A 31-year-old primigravida at 36 weeks' gestation presents with a blood pressure of 170/110 mmHg, proteinuria, persistent headache and hyperreflexia. She requires delivery by lower segment caesarean section (LSCS) within three hours. Justify your choice of anaesthesia for caesarean section.

This patient has severe pre-eclampsia and her condition requires simultaneous assessment and management as it presents a medical/obstetric emergency.

My choice of anaesthesia would be an epidural at level L1–L2 with 0.5% bupivacaine topped up slowly to a level of dermatome T4 block.

Justification of choice
1. The three hours allows slow establishment of the block.
2. The epidural avoids the complications of general anaesthetic, including:
   - a difficult airway of a pregnant patient exacerbated by upper-airway oedema of pregnancy-induced hypertension (PIH)
   - the risk of regurgitation during intubation/extubation
   - sudden sympathetic surge during direct laryngoscopy that may cause cerebral stroke, sudden myocardial ischaemia and decreased uteroplacental blood flow.
3. It minimises the risk of cardiorespiratory and uteroplacental suppression by volatile anaesthetic agents.
4. It prevents the risk of awareness during LSCS.

Benefits of epidural in this case
The benefits here outweigh the risks. They are:
- good intraoperative conditions
- good postoperative analgesia
- sympathetic block attenuating blood pressure rise during surgical stress
- facilitates intraoperative blood pressure control
- allows for mother–baby bonding to start early
- conscious-state monitoring during LSCS, allowing for vigilance for eclamptic fit.

Risks of epidural in this case
1. It is a difficult technique. Multiple attempts cause dural puncture leading to an increased risk of postdural puncture headache.
2. Coagulopathy developing intraoperatively increases the risk of epidural haematoma.

3. Sympathetic block may complicate the degree of hypovolaemic shock from massive bleeding intraoperatively.
4. A high thoracic block may impair chest compliance and increase the work of breathing.

Further reading

Barker P, Callender CC. Coagulation screening before epidural analgesia in pre-eclampsia. *Anaesthesia* 1991; **46**:64–7.

Buchan AS, McCrae AF. Epidural and spinal analgesia in obstetrics. *Curr Opin Anesthesiol* 1992; **5**:329–32.

Carrie LES. Spinal and/or epidural blockade for caesarian section. In: Reynolds F (ed.), *Epidural and Spinal Blockade in Obstetrics*. London: Ballière Tindall, 1990, pp. 139–50.

2 Control of blood pressure in pre-eclampsia

> A 31-year-old primigravida at 36 weeks' gestation presents with a blood pressure of 170/110mmHg, proteinuria, persistent headache and hyperreflexia. She requires delivery by lower segment caesarean section (LSCS) within three hours. How would you manage her blood pressure in the time before surgery?

This patient has severe pre-eclampsia and her condition requires simultaneous assessment and management as it presents a medical/obstetric emergency.

Assessment

1. *History and examination* looking for problems associated with multisystem involvement that occurs with pregnancy-induced hypertension (PIH) – already elicited in the question.
2. *Neurological:* fitting, increased irritability, hypertensive bleed.
3. *Renal:* oliguria, acute tubular necrosis, proteinuria.
4. *Cardiovascular:* decreased blood volume, vasoconstriction, raised blood pressure (BP).
5. *Hepatic:* abnormal liver function tests.
6. *Respiratory:* pulmonary oedema.
7. *Haematological:* haemolysis, thrombocytopenia.
8. *Fetal:* decreased placental blood flow, abruption, growth retardation.

Investigations with placement of intravenous (IV) cannula

1. Large bore IV cannula.
2. Serum electrolytes.
3. Uric acid level.
4. Liver fuction tests.
5. Full blood count – platelet count may be low.
6. Cross-match/or group and save.
7. Placement of urinary catheter.
8. Placement of invasive arterial BP monitoring if available or transfer to area where possible.

Hypotensive agents

Institute IV fluid rehydration alongside vasodilators: a 500-mL bolus of normal saline, then 1–1.5mL/kg/min. Aim for MAP of 105–130mmHg. **Do not drop BP precipitously.**

Agents

1. Hydralazine 5 mg IV every 10–15 minutes – acts within 10–15 minutes and lasts 20–30 minutes.
2. Sodium nitroprusside infusion starting at 1 μg/kg/min – requires invasive monitoring.
3. Magnesium sulphate may be used to lower blood pressure as well as for prophylaxis against convulsions because it acts as a vasodilator. The dose is 4 Gm IV bolus over 20 minutes, then infusion 2–4 Gm/HR hour.

Starting the epidural

When the platelet count comes back within normal range and the blood pressure and fluid volume status are under better control, insert and start the epidural block. Use 3–5 mL bolus of 0.5% bupivacaine plain. Slow titration is needed.

Keep checking the block and BP. Apply fluid load as required, and top up the epidural as required.

Further reading

Benhamou D. Complications of obstetric anaesthesia. *Curr Opin Anaesthesiol* 1995; 8:216–19.

Howell PR, Rubin AP. Pre-eclampsia, eclampsia and the anaesthetist. *Curr Anaesth Crit Care* 1991; **2**:101–7.

Morgan BM. Pregnancy, hypertension and pre-eclampsia. *Curr Opin Anesthesiol* 1994; 7:231–9.

3   Control of pre-eclamptic convulsions

> A 31-year-old primigravida delivered a healthy child by caesarian section at 36 weeks' gestation. She presented with a blood pressure of 170/110mmHg, protein-uria, persistent headache and hyperreflexia. She had an uneventful general anaesthetic, but started convulsing in the recovery ward two hours postoperatively. How would you manage this?

This is a life-threatening situation and assessment, diagnosis and management need to proceed urgently and simultaneously. Fits range from partial to generalised and may not be sustained.

First actions

The priority is to prevent the woman injuring herself, so avoid manipulating her airway until the fit is over. If the fit is ongoing, use an anticonvulsant – diazepam 10 mg IV – as soon as possible. Put her in the left lateral position with head down. Give high-flow oxygen via a facemask.

Following actions

Check the airway for breathing and circulation. If the woman's condition is unstable with regard to her ventilation and airway, she should be sedated and a rapid-sequence intubation performed – then ventilate her while stabilising her haemodynamically (fluids IV and monitoring). Suitable drugs are:
* diazepam 10 mg IV
* thiopentone 50 mg IV
* suxamethonium 100 mg IV.

Look for an obvious cause

The most obvious cause would be her eclampsia, but exclude:
* hypoxia/hypercarbia
* electrolyte abnormalities – hypo- or hypercalcaemia
* hypomagnesaemia
* hypo- or hypernatraemia (syntocinon)
    * – go through a systematic approach – cover abcd – 'a swift check'.
* hypoglycaemia.

Further management
1. Optimise physiological and biochemical variables.
2. Ensure adequate anticonvulsants:
    magnesium sulphate infusion
    phenytoin 15 mg/kg at 50 mg/min IV.

3. Consult with the gynaecologist/obstetrician.
4. Arrange an ICU bed and appropriate follow-up care.

Further reading

Benhamou D. Complications of obstetric anaesthesia. *Curr Opin Anesthesiol* 1995; **8**:216–19.

Howell PR, Rubin AP. Pre-eclampsia, eclampsia and the anaesthetist. *Curr Anaesth Crit Care* 1991; **2**:101–7.

Miles JF, Martin JN, Blake PG *et al*. Post-partum eclampsia: a recurring perinatal dilemma. *Obstet Gynaecol* 1990; **76**:328–31.

Morgan BM. Pregnancy, hypertension and pre-eclampsia. *Curr Opin Anesthesiol* 1994; **7**:231–9.

4 Repeat caesarean section

A 34-year-old woman requires repeat lower-section caesarean section (LSCS). Last time she had a caesarean section her postoperative course was complicated by postdural puncture headache (following dural puncture with a 16-gauge needle), as well as a deep venous thrombosis. She refuses general anaesthesia. Explain the regional anaesthesia technique you have chosen.

In the absence of contradiction of the technique, I would select a spinal anaesthetic with a small-gauge pencil-point needle (ideally a 27-gauge Whitacre needle). I would use approximately 2.4–2.6 mL of bupivacaine (heavy) along with 200 µg of morphine with a 1000–1500-mL crystalloid preload. I would follow this by testing the sensory block and managing haemodynamics as appropriate, with monitoring of respiratory function up to 24 hours postoperatively.

Advantages of this technique
1. It is a reliable block with rapid onset and good intraoperative analgesia.
2. There is a lower incidence of postdural puncture headache with the needle selected.
3. A regional technique is associated with reduced maternal morbidity/mortality for LSCS.
4. Bupivacaine (heavy) allows some control over the height of the block along with reduced duration of motor block compared to plain solution.
5. Morphine provides up to 16 hours of analgesia which may aid her in early mobilisation (possibly the most important prevention for DVT).
6. There are low incidences of critical side-effects (late respiratory depression).
7. Respiratory depression requires appropriate postoperative monitoring, especially of sedation scores and respiratory rate/S_pO2.
8. Other side-effects of morphine (e.g. pruritus/nausea and vomiting), while common, can usually be treated.

Further reading
Morgan M. Obstetric anaesthesia and analgesia. In: Nimmo WS, Rowbotham DJ, Smith G (eds), *Anaesthesia*, 2nd edn. Oxford: Blackwell Scientific, 1994, pp. 1000–28.
Stackhouse RA, Hughes SC. Caesarian section. *Curr Opin Anaesthesiol* 1994; 7:231–9.

5 Prophylaxis for deep vein thrombosis (DVT)

> A 34-year-old woman requires repeat lower-section caesarean section LSCS). Last time she had a caesarean section her postoperative course was complicated by postdural puncture headache (following dural puncture with a 16-gauge needle), as well as a deep venous thrombosis (DVT). She refuses to have general anaesthesia. Describe and justify your prophylaxis against deep venous thrombosis for her.

DVT prophylaxis: spinal technique

I would refer the patient to a haematologist preoperatively, in particular looking for congenital causes of intravascular thrombosis.

Preoperative factors
1. Not confined to bed.
2. Ambulation prior to theatre.
3. TED (full length) stockings when immobile.
4. Consider subcutaneous unfractionated heparin (e.g. 5000 units b.d.).
5. Fluid hydration whilst fasting.

Perioperative factors
1. Calf compressors prior to establishing block.
2. Fluid hydration prior to establishing block.
3. Timing of procedure prior to next dose of herapin to maximise coagulation for regional technique.

Postoperative factors
1. Continue active calf compressors (sequential) until mobilising.
2. Regular subcutaneous heparin.
3. Early mobilisation and ambulation when block has worn off.
4. Maximise fluid intake and add IV fluids if there is any suggestion of intravascular depletion (e.g. urine output under 1 mL/kg).

Further reading
McKenzie PJ. Anaesthesia and the prophylaxis of thromboembolic diseases. *Curr Anaesth Crit Care* 1993; 4:26–30.

6 Postdural puncture headache

A 34-year-old woman requires repeat lower section caesarean section (LSCS). Last time she had a caesarean section her postoperative course was complicated by postdural puncture headache (following dural puncture with a 16-gauge needle), as well as a deep venous thrombosis. She refuses general anaesthesia. How would you minimise the problem of postdural puncture headache on this occasion?

Minimising postdural puncture headache (PDPH)

Regional anaesthesia options for LSCS
These include:
- epidural
- spinal
- combined epidural/spinal.

Minimising the risk of repeat PDPH
1. See the patient before the operation. Assess the severity of headache/treatment required, and try to ascertain any factors contributing to the earlier dural puncture (e.g. emergency procedure, patient in labour, inexperienced operator, back pathology, ?obese).
2. Discuss with the patient the options and obtain consent (understanding risk of repeat PDPH).
3. If there was difficulty in finding space, it may be reasonable to perform a spinal. The incidence of PDPH with a 25-gauge pencil-point needle is approximately 1.1%, which is comparable with an epidural. However, if it is difficult to locate the epidural space then the incidence may be higher with epidural analgesia.
4. To decrease the risk of dural puncture with epidural analgesia, several precautions can be taken:
   Place the patient in the sitting position.
   Use a smaller-gauge epidural needle (e.g 18).
   Align the bevel parallel with fibres.
   Use saline for loss of resistance.
5. Follow the patient up and ask the nursing staff to make contact if headache develops.
   If the puncture occurred at the time of needle insertion, then:
   1. Treat conservatively with analgesics and hydration, and prevent constipation.

2. Perform a blood patch if the headache is not settling within 24 hours.
3. Run an epidural infusion for postoperative pain (may decrease the incidence of headache).

Further reading

Bergqvist D, Lindblad B, Matzsch T. Low-molecular-weight heparin for thromboprophylaxis and epidural/spinal anaesthesia: is there a risk? *Acta Anaesth Scand* 1992; **36**:605–9.

Carrie LES. Postdural puncture headache and extradural blood patch. *Br J Anaesth* 1993; **71**:179–80 (editorial).

Carson DF, Serpell MG. Clinical characteristics of commonly used spinal needles. *Anaesthesia* 1995; **50**:523–5.

Multiple-choice questions: Obstetrics

1. Ritodrine can cause:
   a) bradycardia
   b) heart block
   c) left ventricular failure
   d) hypotension
   e) peripheral vasconstriction.

2. Infant respiratory distress syndrome:
   a) usually occurs within 12 hours of delivery
   b) usually occurs after caesarean section
   c) has a better prognosis if steroids are given to the infant
   d) is uncommon after 36 weeks' gestation
   e) is more common in multiple pregnancies.

3. The second twin becomes 'stuck' following the administration of ergometrine. The following drugs will reliably relax the uterus:
   a) thiopentone
   b) suxamethonium
   c) ritodrine
   d) salbutamol
   e) halothane.

4. The idiopathic respiratory distress syndrome:
   a) occurs 12 hours after delivery
   b) is more common following caesarean section
   c) is caused by lack of surfactant
   d) is more common in babies delivered post-term
   e) presents with cyanosis.

5. For caesarean section under epidural:
   a) never give more that 20 mL of 0.5% bupivacaine
   b) the block must extend from T5 to S1
   c) you must give syntocinon rather than ergometrine
   d) you must also do a paracervical block
   e) you should preload with 500 mL of Hartmann's solution.

6. You are asked to provide anaesthesia for a patient with a breech delivery
   when difficulty is being experienced with the fetal head. The following are
   acceptable techniques:
   a) spinal
   b) epidural
   c) cyclopropane
   d) thiopentone, suxamethonium, intubation
   e) ketamine.

7. In a pregnant woman at term:
   a) tidal volume is increased
   b) functional residual capacity is increased
   c) physiological dead-space is decreased
   d) total vital capacity is reduced
   e) airway resistance is reduced.
8. Amniotic fluid embolism can cause:
   a) bronchospasm
   b) bleeding
   c) peripheral cyanosis
   d) pulmonary hypertension
   e) hypertension.
9. Diazoxide is used in the treatment of pre-eclampsia because:
   a) it causes a diuresis
   b) given intravenously it causes hypotension
   c) it prevents hypoglycaemia
   d) it increases uterine contractility
   e) it provides useful sedation.
10. Pethidine is used in obstetrics because:
    a) it is 75% excreted unchanged
    b) it does not cross the placenta
    c) it causes less respiratory depression than an equipotent dose of morphine
    d) it can be used without medical supervision
    e) it does not affect uterine contractility.
11. In the management of uterine haemorrhage the following are used:
    a) IV fibrinogen
    b) IV ergometrine
    c) aortic compression
    d) uterine packing
    e) bimanual compression.
12. Causes of a low Apgar score (<5) following lower-segment caesarean section (LSCS) are:
    a) maternal hypoxia
    b) uterine incision-delivery time greater than 90 s
    c) placental transfer of muscle relaxant
    d) reduced uterine contractility
    e) reduced placental blood flow.

13. Suxamethonium does not cross the placenta because of:
    a) placental cholinesterase
    b) high protein binding
    c) it being an elongated molecule
    d) its high degree of ionization
    e) insufficient maternal concentration.
14. Signs of fetal distress include:
    a) loss of beat to beat variation
    b) transverse lie
    c) fetal respiratory movements
    d) early decelerations
    e) late decelerations.
15. In the fetal transfer of drugs given by the epidural route:
    a) the placenta is an effective barrier
    b) fetal bradycardia may occur with local analgesics
    c) highly protein-bound drugs are transferred less
    d) amide-linked local analgesics should be avoided
    e) opiates should be avoided.
16. A pregnant mother at term:
    a) has increased gastric tone
    b) may develop hypotension if turned on her side
    c) has an increased cardiac output (compared with non-pregnant state)
    d) has decreased vital capacity
    e) has decreased MAC for inhalational agents.
17. Amniotic fluid embolism:
    a) can occur during therapeutic abortion
    b) occurs only following delivery
    c) may present as haemorrhage
    d) definitive diagnosis can be made only at post-mortem
    e) is more common in multiparous women.
18. Apgar score:
    a) is of no value in caesarean sections
    b) is made one minute after delivery of the head
    c) heart rate is of more use than colour
    d) cannot be applied to coloured babies
    e) is a sensitive index of neonatal depression.
19. Anti-D antibodies that develop in a rhesus-negative mother with a rhesus-positive child:
    a) cause anaemia in the fetus
    b) cause jaundice in the fetus
    c) fetal rbc are found in maternal circulation
    d) occurs during the first trimester only
    e) develop because of antigen crossing the placenta.

Answers to multiple-choice questions

	a)	b)	c)	d)	e)
1.	a) False;	b) False;	c) True;	d) True;	e) False
2.	a) True;	b) False;	c) False;	d) True;	e) True
3.	a) False;	b) False;	c) False;	d) False;	e) True
4.	a) False;	b) True;	c) True;	d) False;	e) False
5.	a) False;	b) False;	c) True;	d) False;	e) False
6.	a) False;	b) False;	c) False;	d) True;	e) False
7.	a) True;	b) False;	c) True;	d) True;	e) False
8.	a) False;	b) True;	c) True;	d) True;	e) False
9.	a) True;	b) True;	c) True;	d) False;	e) False
10.	a) False;	b) False;	c) False;	d) True;	e) True
11.	a) False;	b) True;	c) True;	d) True;	e) True
12.	a) True;	b) True;	c) False;	d) False;	e) True
13.	a) False;	b) False;	c) False;	d) True;	e) False
14.	a) True;	b) False;	c) False;	d) False;	e) True
15.	a) False;	b) True;	c) False;	d) False;	e) False
16.	a) False;	b) False;	c) True;	d) True;	e) True
17.	a) True;	b) False;	c) True;	d) False;	e) True
18.	a) False;	b) True;	c) True;	d) False;	e) False
19.	a) True;	b) True;	c) True;	d) False;	e) True

Answers to multiple-choice questions

PAEDIATRIC ANAESTHESIA

1 Latex allergy

> A 9-year-old child with spina bifida presenting for a tendon transfer procedure has latex allergy. What precautions should be taken perioperatively to prevent this child developing a latex reaction? What advice do you give the parents?

Latex has increasingly been recognised as an important cause of allergic reactions. The prevalence in a general population with no specific risk factors is thought to be less than 1%. Reactions may occur some time after exposure. Latex is found in many articles in everyday life as well as items of medical equipment. A box containing equipment which is safe to use should be readily available.

Preoperative considerations

General
1. Make the patient the first on the operating list.
2. Give no premedication.
3. Remove bins from the theatre.
4. Remove all latex items.
5. Limit staff numbers.
6. Inform all staff.

The anaesthetic machine
1. Use plastic circuits.
2. Use plastic masks.
3. LMA contains silicone and not latex.
4. Use an old, well-washed bag on the breathing circuit.
5. Use a bacteria filter.
6. Use a PVC endotracheal tube.

Monitoring
1. Use tegaderm under saturation probe.
2. Use bandage under an NIBP cuff.

IV equipment
1. Remove bungs and replace with 3-way tap.
2. Use an interlink system made of polypropylene.
3. Draw drugs up just prior to use. Do not leave in syringes for long periods.
4. Do not use multidose vials of drugs.

Intraoperative considerations

1. Use powder-free non-latex gloves.
2. Apply full non-invasive monitoring in accordance with AAGBI guidelines.
3. Check the availability of adrenaline, chlorpheniramine, hydrocortisone, fluids, lines, defibrillation, experienced help.

Postoperative considerations

1. Apply similar precautions in recovery.
2. Discharge from hospital as soon as feasible.

Advice to parents

- The presentation of latex allergy can be very variable, from rash through to life-threatening reactions involving lung and cardiovascular dysfunction.
- Latex allergy is a well-recognised condition and their child has significant risk factors.
- Despite all efforts to remove latex products from the perioperative period, latex reactions will still occur in <5% of patients.
- Latex allergy can be treated with adrenaline, IV fluids and supportive measures with a good prognosis. There is, however, still a mortality rate of 15% if the child develops anaphylaxis despite the best efforts being made.

Further reading

Association of Anaesthetists. *Anaphylactic Reactions Associated with Anaesthesia*. London: AA, 1998.

Dakin MJ, Yentis SM. Latex allergy: a strategy for management. *Anaesthesia* 1998; **53**:774–81.

Health and Safety Executive. *Latex and You*. London: Health & Safety Executive document INDG 320, May 2000; www.hse.gov.uk.

Wildsmith JAW, McKinnon RP. Histaminoid reactions in anaesthesia. *Br J Anaesth* 1995; **74**:217–28.

2 Investigation of latex allergy

A 9-year-old child with spina bifida presenting for a tendon transfer procedure is said to have multiple allergies including latex and antibiotics. How would you investigate whether this child does have latex allergy?

Latex exposure can occur via a number of routes such as airborne, intravenous and mucosal exposure. There is evidence that repeated exposure over time increases the incidence of sensitivity. The various chemicals added during processing of latex can provoke an irritant dermatitis which is not an allergic reaction. Some reactions may be due to a type IV hypersensitivity contact dermatitis, developing 24–48 hours after exposure. These are thought to be provoked by the chemicals added during rubber production and are mediated by T-lymphocytes. Of more concern are type I immediate hypersensitivity reactions ranging from urticarial skin rashes to full-blown anaphylaxis. Type I reactions mediated by IgE antibody to latex protein antigens result in mast cell degranulation with the release of mediators such as histamine, tryptase, prostaglandins and leukotrienes.

The manifestation will vary depending on the area of application. Reaction on the skin is as *urticarial rash*. Mucosal exposure to latex can lead to clinical *anaphylaxis*.

History and examination

This child already has several risk factors such as spina bifida and allergy to antibiotics.

- Obtain a history from old hospital notes. Has the child had formal testing?
- The prevalence of latex allergy in patients with spina bifida has been reported as 60%, thought to be due to repeated bladder catheterisation.
- Take a careful history of symptoms and signs of possible previous allergic reaction to latex: skin reaction, bronchospasm, anaphylaxis, previous supportive treatment (e.g ICU treatment).
- Multiple operations, especially laparotomies, are a risk factor.
- Other risk factors are allergy to fruit, nuts, balloons and atopy.
- Look for evidence of dermatitis, although this can be caused by several mechanisms and is clinically difficult to distinguish.

Investigations

Patients with suspected latex allergy should be tested by an experienced centre. The initial investigation is a radio-allergosorbent test (RAST) for IgE. This involves the reaction of the patient's serum with an antigen polymer complex in the presence of [125I]-labelled IgE antibody. This allows quantification of the amount of antibody present in the patient's serum. The rate of false negative results is approximately 20%.

If the RAST is negative and a strong clinical history is present, then proceed to skin-prick testing with a needle. This is carried out with a latex antigen solution at a variety of dilutions, with full resuscitative equipment and monitoring. A wheal indicates a positive test.

As none of these methods are infallible, a patient with a strongly suggestive history but negative tests should be managed as though latex-sensitive.

Further reading

Watkins J. Investigations of allergic and hypersensitivity reactions to anaesthetic agents. *Br J Anaesth* 1987; **59**:104–11.

Wildsmith JAW, McKinnon RP. Histaminoid reactions in anaesthesia. *Br J Anaesth* 1995; **74**:217–28.

3 Paediatric pain

What are the choices for postoperative analgesia for a child aged 4 years presenting for repair of an inguinal hernia as a day case? State briefly the advantages and
disadvantages of each method.

The choices are as follows:
1. *Non-local anaesthetic techniques*
        rectal route: paracetamol, NSAIDs
        opiates.
    Local anaesthetic techniques
        caudal
        nerve block
        local infiltration.

Discussion

Analgesia for children should provide subjective comfort by inhibition of
trauma-induced nociception to allow early restoration of normal life particularly in the day-case setting. A multi-model approach with simultaneous
administration of analgesics which work by different mechanisms has the
advantage of alternating nociceptive impulses at various sites, thereby allowing
the use of smaller doses of each drug, minimising side-effects.

There can be very few operations in children where the quality of analgesia
is not enhanced by concomitant use of paracetamol with or without a non-
steroid anti-inflammatory drug (NSAID). Paracetamol is presented in a wide
range of formulations, and suppositories are an increasingly popular route for
minor analgesic medication in children, especially whilst the patient is under
general anaesthesia. The use of suppositories should be discussed beforehand
with the parents. The initial analgesic dose of paracetamol when given by the
rectal route is 20–30 mg/kg, and 20 mg/kg per 6 hours thereafter. Paracetamol's
antipyretic properties are useful in controlling postoperative malaise due to
temperature.

There are three NSAIDs that are useful in paediatric postoperative analgesia: ibuprofen, diclofenac and ketorolac. Only ibuprofen suspension is
licensed for pain relief in children over the age of 1 year. All three are commonly
used for postoperative analgesia, however. NSAIDs may be used in children with
asthma, but *if there is any deterioration in respiratory status they must be stopped
immediately*. NSAIDs should be given in the minimum effective dose.

Single-shot caudal extradural analgesia has been widely used in paediatric
anaesthesia for many years. Plain bupivacaine 0.25% at a dose of 0.5 mL/kg is
given for low thoracic blocks. Local anaesthetic toxicity is rare in single-shot

caudals. Short, bevelled needles should be used as these are less likely to puncture epidural veins. Unlike in adults, test doses of local anaesthetic with adrenaline (15 mg) do not produce consistent rises in heart rate in anaesthetised children. Thus the total dose of local anaesthetic should be administered slowly in small increments. Single-shot blocks are short-lived, however, and other analgesia must be provided, particularly in the day-case setting.

Caudal extradural opioid given as a single shot is not recommended in day-case anaesthesia because of the high incidence of side-effects, namely pruritus, urinary retention, nausea and vomiting.

Ilioinguinal and iliohypogastric nerve blocks can be performed for unilateral hernia repair. The advantage of this technique is that anatomical landmarks are often clearer in children than in adults. In experienced hands this is a safe, reliable technique with a low failure rate.

Local anaesthetic infiltration around the incision by the surgeon can also provide effective pain relief. Bupivacaine is the local anaesthetic of choice owing to its longer action.

If a local anaesthetic block cannot be performed, or if it is unsuccessful, a parenteral narcotic such as fentanyl 1–2 µg/kg should be administered intraoperatively. Nausea, vomiting, dysphoria, respiratory depression and prolonged sedation – all of which will delay discharge – are potential side-effects. Procedures requiring repeated administration of narcotic analgesics are unsuitable for day-case surgery.

Further reading

Armitage EN. Caudal block in children. *Anaesthesia* 1979; **34**:396.

Arthur DS, McNicol LR. Local anaesthetic techniques in paediatric surgery. *Br J Anaesth* 1986; **58**:760–78.

Casey W, Rice L, Hannallah R *et al.*. A comparison between bupivicaine instillation versus ilioinguinal/iliohypogastric nerve block for postoperative analgesia following inguinal hermiorrhaphy in children. *Anaesthesiology* 1990; **71**:637–9.

Gaudreault P, Guay J, Nicol O, Dupuis C. Pharmacokinetics and clinical efficacy of intra-rectal solutions of acetaminophen. *Can J Anaesth* 1988; **35**:149–52.

Kehlet H. Postoperative pain relief: what is the issue? *Br J Anaesth* 1994; **72**:375–8.

Lloyd-Thomas AR, Howard RF. A pain service for children. *Paediatr Anaesth* 1994; **4**:85–104.

Maunuksesla E-L, Kokki H, Bullingham RES. Comparison of intravenous ketorolac with morphine for postoperative pain in children. *Clin Pharmacol Ther* 1992; **52**:436–43.

4 Premedicant drugs

> Evaluate the use of premedicating drugs before general anaesthesia in a 4-year-old child.

Premedication is often avoided in day-case surgery because of the potential for delayed recovery. Adequate psychological preparation of the child and parent is the singular most important aspect of preoperative preparation. This usually obviates the need for pharmacological premedication.

The child should be prepared for theatre in a calm environment. It is very important to attempt to develop a rapport with any child prior to anaesthesia. This may not be possible in uncooperative children, especially in the very young.

Potential benefits of pharmacological premedication

These include:
* anxiolysis
* sedation
* amnesia
* facilitation of induction of anaesthesia
* postoperative analgesia
* vagolysis
* antiemesis
* anti-sialogogue effect.

These effects must be balanced against the potential unwanted effects such as:
* administration problems
* dysphoria
* cardiorespiratory depression
* nausea/vomiting
* restlessness
* pruritus
* dizziness
* delayed awakening.

Agents

There is a wide range of premedication drugs available which can be administered by many different routes. They include:

1. *trimeprazine tartrate* – 3–4 mg/kg orally, 90 minutes preoperatively
2. *midazolam* – 0.5 mg/kg orally, 30 minutes preoperatively
3. *temazepam* – 0.4 mg/kg orally, 60 minutes preoperatively
4. *diazepam* – 0.4 mg/kg orally, 90 minutes preoperatively

5. *hyoscine* – 0.008 mg/kg
6. *chloral hydrate* – 30 mg/kg orally, 90 minutes preoperatively
7. *atropine* – 0.02 mg/kg IM, 45 minutes preoperatively; or 0.04 mg/kg orally, 60 minutes preoperatively.

Discussion

The oral route is normally preferred by the patient, parents and nursing staff. Absorption and the effect of orally administered drugs are often variable, and timing of administration is very important. Intramuscular injections should be avoided.

Opioids provide useful sedation and postoperative analgesia. However, they cause a high incidence of postoperative nausea, vomiting and pruritus. There is little, if any, place for preoperative intramuscular opioids in paediatric anaesthesia. Alternative routes include oral, intranasal, transdermal and transmucosal routes.

Benzodiazepines have a wide therapeutic index and side-effects are rare. Oral midazolam is unpalatable unless mixed with a small volume of squash drink.

Trimeprazine can provide effective sedation and anxiolysis, and has useful antiemetic properties, but its prolongation of waking time makes it unsuitable in day-case anaesthesia.

Oral chloral hydrate and rectal methohexitone are effective but limited in the setting of day-case anaesthesia by their prolonged effect.

Anticholinergic drugs are routinely used by some anaesthetists to reduce airway irritability, avoid reflex bradycardias and preserve the heart rate during inhalational induction. Others reserve their use for certain indications such as repeated suxamethonium, ocular surgery and bradyarrhythmias. Atropine can be given effectively via the oral or rectal routes.

Special cases

In uncooperative, terrified children who refuse an intravenous injection and a facemask, intramuscular ketamine 2 mg/kg may be useful.

If an intravenous induction technique is planned, Ametop® or Emla® local anaesthetic creams should be applied over a suitable vein. Ametop® may have certain advantages over Emla®, with a faster onset without causing venoconstriction. It is, however, more expensive than Emla.

Further reading

Booker PD. Premedication. *Curr Opin Anaesthesiol* 1991; **4**:363–6.

Meakin G, Dingwall AE, Addison GM. Effects of fasting and oral premedication on the pH and volume of gastric aspirate in children. *Br J Anaesth* 1987; **59**:678–82.

Van der Walt JH, Nicholls B, Bentley M, Tomkins DP. Oral premedication in children. *Anaesth Intens Care* 1987; **15**:151–7.

5 Sevoflurane versus propofol

Compare propofol with sevoflurane as the sole general anaesthesia agent for a 3-year-old child requiring insertion of drainage tubes for chronic otitis media.

The anaesthetic requirements for this operation are:
* smooth induction
* akinesia during insertion of tubes
* rapid return of consciousness as patients are usually day cases.

Both sevoflurane and propofol can deliver a satisfactory anaesthetic for this operation.

Propofol

Advantages
1. Rapid, smooth induction.
2. Ability to titrate depth of anaesthesia in spontaneously ventilating patients using an infusion pump.
3. Rapid recovery.
4. Low incidence of postoperative nausea and vomiting (PONV).

Disadvantages
1. IV access required.
2. Pain on injection.
3. Fewer anaesthetists familiar with total intravenous anaesthesia for 3-year-old patients.
4. Not licensed for use in young children in some countries.

Sevoflurane

Advantages
1. Rapid smooth induction (smells pleasant, low blood/gas solubility coefficient).
2. Avoidance of IV access prior to anaesthesia.
3. Easy to titrate depth of anaesthesia with end-tidal concentration (easier than with propofol).
4. Rapid recovery possible.
5. Cheaper than propofol.

Disadvantages
1. Child may find gas induction unacceptable.
2. Child may display very agitated behaviour for 5–10 minutes after recovery (more common with sevoflurane than other volatile anaesthetic agents).
3. Perhaps a higher PONV rate due to lack of antiemetic effect of propofol.

Further reading

Meakin G. Drugs in paediatric anaesthesia. *Curr Opin Anaesthesiol* 1994; **7**:251–6.

Proctor LT, Gregory GA. Paediatric anaesthesia. *Curr Opin Anaesthesiol* 1995; **8**:221–56.

Strunin L. How long should patients fast before surgery? Time for new guidelines. *Br J Anaesth* 1993; **70**:1–3.

6 Tracheo-oesophageal fistula repair

Describe the anaesthetic management of a neonate requiring tracheo-oesophageal fistula repair.

Tracheo-oesophageal fistula (TOF) and oesophageal atresia, without prenatal screening, has an incidence of 1 in 3000–3500 live births. This incidence is falling in countries that undertake prenatal screening initially using ultrasound, and then by amniocentesis. With careful and skilled anaesthetic and surgical management, the survival rate in babies with no other abnormalities approaches 100%. The overall mortality is 10–15%. The most common presentation is the combination of oesophageal atresia with a fistula between the distal trachea and the lower part of the oesophagus.

Preoperative assessment

Many infants are of low birthweight and approximately 30% are premature. There are frequent difficulties with feeding from the outset, and the baby is often noted to have copious upper-airway secretions owing to an inability to swallow. Attempts at passing a nasogastric tube are unsuccessful. Coughing, choking and cyanosis occur if feeding is attempted. A plain radiograph will demonstrate a coiled radio-opaque tube in the oesophageal pouch. A gas bubble in the stomach confirms the presence of a lower pouch fistula. Total absence of air in the abdomen on the radiograph usually indicates pure oesophageal atresia without TOF. Barium studies are contraindicated because of the risk of pulmonary aspiration.

There is a high incidence of associated abnormalities (at least 50%) and a thorough examination of the baby must be carried out, augmented with appropriate investigations. The most common associated anomalies are imperforate anus, small bowel atresia, and skeletal, urogenital and cardiac abnormalities. The VATER syndrome consists of vertebral, anorectal, TOF, renal, radial and rib abnormalities. All babies should have an echocardiogram to exclude cardiac pathology which is present in 25%.

From the moment of birth the baby is at risk of aspirating saliva, feeds and gastric contents via the communicating fistula. The contents of the upper oesophageal pouch should be isolated from the lungs and continuously aspirated with a Replogle tube. In an otherwise uncomplicated case, pulmonary aspiration poses the greatest risk to postoperative survival. An assessment should be made of any lung soiling from aspiration, by clinical and radiological examination of the chest. The operation should be delayed if there has been significant aspiration with evidence of collapse/consolidation of one or more lobes. Antibiotics and physiotherapy should be commenced. Otherwise the operation is usually performed on the same day.

Preoperatively the baby should be nursed prone and slightly head-down to aid drainage of the secretions. When effective drainage of the upper pouch has been ensured, the baby can be nursed in a head-up position to minimize reflux of gastric contents through a distal TOF. Occasionally, the baby will require preoperative intubation and ventilation.

Routine preoperative investigations include a full blood count, urea and electrolytes, blood glucose, arterial or capillary blood gases, and a chest radiograph.

Anaesthetic technique

It is imperative that the baby's heat losses be minimized. This is best achieved with a warm operating theatre (25°C), a thermostatically controlled air mattress, humidification of inspired gases, and silver foil wrapped around all exposed parts, especially the head.

Monitoring should consist routinely of electrocardiography (ECG), blood pressure, pulse oximetry, core temperature and precordial stethoscope. An arterial line may be *in situ* if the baby has undergone preoperative assisted ventilation, or can be sited intraoperatively, if postoperative ventilation is anticipated; otherwise non-invasive measurement of blood pressure is satisfactory.

An intravenous cannula will already have been sited. Anaesthesia is induced and maintained subsequently with nitrous oxide and inhalational agent (sevoflurane 1–2% or 0.5% isoflurane) in oxygen. Atracurium 0.5 mg/kg produces muscle relaxation for controlled ventilation. An endotracheal tube of 2.5 mm or 3.0 mm will be required. The position of the endotracheal tube is crucial, as malpositioning runs the risk of distending the stomach and underventilating the lungs. Auscultation over the stomach and lung fields will confirm correct placement of the endotracheal tube (i.e. good air entry into both lung fields with minimal gastric inflation). It is very important to note the length of the tube at the mouth, and to ensure its reliable fixation.

Intraoperative analgesia can be provided with a short-acting narcotic such as fentanyl 2 μg/kg. Larger doses may be given if postoperative controlled ventilation is planned. Controlled ventilation should be performed manually, so that any changes in the patency of the tube, or inflating pressure, due to surgical retraction or blood are detected immediately. Continuous auscultation over the lung fields will detect a change in position of the endotracheal tube which may compromise ventilation.

All intravenous fluids must be warmed. Blood loss is not usually heavy, but the evaporative losses consequent on thoracotomy are considerable. Blood transfusion should be initiated if blood loss exceeds 10% of the estimated circulating blood volume (the circulating blood volume is 80–100 mL/kg). All intravenous fluids should be administered with a syringe to ensure accurate volume replacement. Muscle relaxation is reversed with neostigmine and atropine, and the trachea is extubated with the baby awake.

Postoperative management

Further postoperative analgesia can be provided by local infiltration of local anaesthetic into the muscles and skin wound (bupivacaine, up to 2 mg/kg). Postoperative ventilation is indicated only if the anastomosis is under significant tension or if the status of the patient was poor preoperatively (very low birthweight, significant cardiac anomaly, aspiration). Postoperative sedation, paralysis and controlled ventilation are continued for 5 days. Nutrition is provided intravenously, or enterally via a nasogastric tube or gastrotomy.

Preterm babies display increased sensitivity to anaesthetic agents and great care must be exercised in administering parenteral narcotics; postoperative observation in a well-staffed neonatal intensive care unit is mandatory. They are at increased risk of postoperative apnoea, with or without narcotics, and they should be nursed on an apnoea mattress.

Intraventricular cerebral haemorrhage occurs in 40–50% of babies less than 35 weeks' postconceptual age. This may result in altered consciousness and respiratory abnormalities in the short term, and may be complicated by neurodevelopmental delay and hydrocephalus later. Preterm babies also have an increased sensitivity to infection.

Further reading

James IG. Emergencies in paediatric anaesthesia. In: Sumner E, Hatch DJ (eds), *Textbook of Paediatric Anaesthesia Practice*, London: Ballière Tindall, 1989.

Spitz L. Complications in the surgery of oesophageal atresia. *Paediatr Surg Int* 1987; **2**:1–2.

Wright VM. Oesophageal atresia. *Br J Hosp Med* 1989; **42**:452–60.

Multiple-choice questions: Paediatric anaesthesia

1. Cyanosis at birth occurs in:
   a) tetralogy of Fallot
   b) transposition of the great vessels
   c) pulmonary stenosis (isolated)
   d) patent ductus arteriosus
   e) ventricular septal defect.

2. Respiratory distress syndrome in the neonate:
   a) is more common after caesarean section
   b) occurs within 12 hours of birth
   c) is treated by intravenous steroids given to the infant
   d) is more common after 36 weeks' gestation
   e) is more common following epidural analgesia in labour.

3. Surfactant:
   a) prevents alveoli collapsing as lung volume decreases
   b) is produced by type II pneumocytes
   c) contains phosphatidyl choline
   d) is reduced in the infant respiratory distress syndrome
   e) increases surface tension.

4. A peanut lodged in a child's bronchus commonly presents with:
   a) haemoptysis
   b) chronic cough
   c) interstitial emphysema
   d) distal lung collapse
   e) empyema.

5. Causes of respiratory distress in the neonate include:
   a) unilateral choanal atresia
   b) tracheo-oesophageal fistula
   c) diaphragmatic hernia
   d) necrotizing enterocolitis
   e) myelomeningocoele.

6. Neonates compared to adults have:
   a) decreased oxygen consumption
   b) decreased ability to shiver
   c) increased V_d/V_t
   d) increased body surface area/weight ratio
   e) increased airway resistance.

7. Recognised causes of stridor in infancy include:
   a) bronchiolitis
   b) tracheomalacia
   c) laryngotracheobronchitis
   d) epiglottitis
   e) laryngomalacia.

8. In an infant with persistent vomiting the following are true:
   a) bile in the vomit supports the diagnosis of duodenal atresia
   b) abdominal x-ray would be useful
   c) no bile supports the diagnosis of pyloric stenosis
   d) duodenal atresia is more likely in Down syndrome
   e) the patient should be rehydrated and the stomach aspirated preoperatively.

9. In epiglottitis the following are true:
   a) IV access should be performed first
   b) immediate lateral neck x-ray will aid diagnosis
   c) IV chloramphenicol is the treatment of choice
   d) tracheostomy should be performed if the patient is still intubated after 72 hours
   e) the patient is likely to be intubated for 5 days.

10. The following are true about the fetal circulation:
   a) the P_aO_2 in the descending aorta is lower than that in the aortic arch
   b) the ductus venosus contains mixed venous blood
   c) the ductus arteriosus closes due to the rise in systemic pressure
   d) closure of the foramen ovale is due to the change in left and right atrial pressures
   e) blood from the inferior vena cava can reach the systemic circulation.

11. Premature neonates:
   a) are prone to hypocalaemia
   b) have decreased insensible losses
   c) have increased type 1 oxidative fibres in the diaphragm
   d) are sensitive to non-depolarising muscle relaxants
   e) are prone to hypothermia.

12. A 4-year-old child with a 4-day history of wheeze unresponsive to nebulised salbutamol and to adrenaline who is cyanosed and restless (P_aO_2 5 kPa, P_aCO_2 10 kPa) should be initially treated with:
   a) intravenous bicarbonate
   b) intravenous aminophylline
   c) immediate intubation and ventilation
   d) intravenous diazepam
   e) sodium cronoglycate.

13. An 8-year-old boy is rescued from water after 20 minutes' immersion. His core temperature is 30°C. Immediate management includes:
   a) hypoventilation
   b) rapid warming
   c) pentobarbitone infusion
   d) cardiopulmonary resuscitation
   e) intravenous steroids.

Answers to multiple-choice questions

1. a) True;   b) True;   c) False;   d) True;   e) False
2. a) True;   b) False;   c) False;   d) False;   e) False
3. a) True;   b) True;   c) True;   d) True;   e) False
4. a) False; b) True;   c) False;   d) True;   e) False
5. a) True;   b) True;   c) True;   d) True;   e) False
6. a) False; b) True;   c) False;   d) True;   e) True
7. a) False; b) True;   c) True;   d) True;   e) True
8. a) False; b) True;   c) True;   d) True;   e) True
9. a) False; b) False; c) True;   d) False;   e) False
10. a) True;   b) True;   c) False;   d) True;   e) True
11. a) True;   b) False; c) False;   d) True;   e) True
12. a) False; b) False; c) True;   d) False;   e) False
13. a) False; b) True;   c) False;   d) True;   e) False

SECTION EIGHT

PAIN MANAGEMENT

1 Measurement of pain

> Describe the methods available for the measurement of pain.

Assessments and comparisons of different forms of therapy and different or new analgesics are made by measurement of pain severity:

Subjective measurement of pain severity:
- Simple word scale.
- Visual analogue scale.
- Measure of pain relief.
- Automatic and semiautomatic systems.
- Pain scores for children.
- Pain-matching techniques.
- Pain-controlled analgesia.
- Differential pain scores.
- McGill pain questionnaire.
- Sensory decision theory.

Objective measurement of pain severity:
- Respiratory changes.
- Biochemical tests.
- Electroencephalography (EEG).

Discussion

The *simple word scale* asks the patient to choose the word which most nearly describes the pain. The four words chosen by Beecher as being least misunderstood were: none, mild, moderate and severe. The six words in the McGill patient pain index are: none, mild, discomforting, distressing, horrible and excruciating. The more words chosen, the greater the sensitivity of distinction but the greater the disagreement of the relative value of the words.

The *visual analogue scale* asks the patient to mark a horizontal or vertical line, usually 10 cm long, according to the severity of the pain. A simple refinement is the pain slide rule whereby the patient moves a cursor and the score is read on the reverse side. The visual analogue scale is simple to operate and easily understood, but reliability is unsatisfactory when the patient is sleepy, fatigued, confused or uncooperative. It has the further disadvantage that it measures the pain score only at the time of assessment.

Instead of assessing the level of pain, the *measure of pain relief* asks the patient to assess the proportional decrease of pain following the administration of analgesics or analgesic procedure.

There are several *automatic and semiautomatic systems*, which have been developed to measure pain. The King's Pain Recorder is a 7-cm 30-segment light-emitting diode (LED) display, which can be illuminated progressively from one end by the patient. At preset intervals the patient's terminal signals ready, and the patient scores the pain by illuminating the display and sends the signal to the recorder. Welchew developed a similar system where the patient moves vertical, slide-type variable resistors, which change an LED display and alter the position of the pen of a pen-recorder. These systems have the advantage that they eliminate observer bias and yield a continuous recording of pain. They do not measure pain during confusion or sleep, however, and by repetitively questioning they concentrate the patient's mind on the pain, possibly increasing the perception of it.

Pain in children may be poorly distinguished from other unpleasant stimuli and situations. Words are replaced by an illustrated scale on which a cursor points variably to a 'happy' or 'unhappy' picture, or the pain can be represented by a pole up which a figure can climb.

When using *pain-matching techniques*, the assessor applies an experimental stimulus until the pain induced matches the pre-existing pain. Pressure, tourniquet ischaemia and radiant heat can be used. The inflicted pain can be measured in units of pressure, time or absorbed energy, and numerical comparisons can be made. However, experimental pain is not entirely comparable because the thresholds of pain are different in intact, undamaged tissues from those in tissues that are inflamed. Furthermore, in comparisons of severe pain some damage of the experimental site is probable and this will, in itself, alter the pain perception.

When using *patient-controlled analgesia*, the patient has control of the amount of analgesic administered within certain limits. The amount of analgesic self-administered should be sufficient to produce pain relief or tolerable discomfort. It is assumed that the amount of drug required to induce this state is proportional to the pain experienced. The advantages of this method are that the method of assessment achieves the goal of treatment, it provides a numerical assessment for statistical analysis, and the patient is not subjected to repeated questioning or disturbance. One disadvantage of this method of assessment is that rates of distribution and elimination of drugs vary from one patient to another, so patients need differing amounts of drug to relieve the same pain. The speed of onset of differential opiates can complicate assessment and the administration of concomitant drugs influences the assessment.

Since there are at least two kinds of pain following most operations – dull pain at rest and sharp pain on movement – *differential pain scores* score these pains separately.

The *McGill pain questionnaire* seeks to provide a global pain assessment by questioning the site, character and severity of the pain, including the relative severity with regard to time, activity and previous experience. It is a useful tool in the management of chronic pain, but it is usually too complex for immediate postoperative use.

The *sensory decision theory* relies on the patient being given pairs of stimuli, which differ in intensity in a random fashion. At least one of the pair is painful to the patient. The number of correctly differentiated signals is an index of the sensitivity of the stimulated area. This method gives a measure of the neurosensory component of pain and the way the sensation is interpreted by the mind.

Since pain is an interpretation of the perceived sensory stimuli, objective measurement of the perception alone is not possible. However, pain engenders pain reaction or pain behaviour. There are *autonomic and biochemical changes*. These changes can be measured by an observer and used in comparisons with other patients who have similar pains from similar sites.

Blood gases, rate of ventilation and changes in lung volumes and capacities all change, particularly following upper abdominal and thoracic surgery. They are not very reproducible or accurate as measures of pain severity when comparing patients who have had similar operations.

Anxiety and other autonomic and hormonal disturbances accompany acute pain. It causes increases in the level of adrenaline, noradrenaline and serotonin, but these increases are also associated with other forms of stress, including venepuncture. There is no correlation between plasma catecholamine concentrations and linear analogue scores of pain in the postoperative period.

A brief painful stimulus produces a detectable evoked potential in a simple two-lead occipitofrontal electroencephalograph (EEG). The height of the cortical deflection is linearly related to the intensity of the stimulus. Nitrous oxide, transcutaneous electrical nerve stimulation (TENS) and acupuncture can reduce the height of this deflection.

Further reading

Chapman CR, Wilson ME, Gehrig JD. Comparative effects of acupuncture and transcutaneous stimulation on the perception of painful dental stimuli. *Pain* 1976; **2**:265–83.

Ready LB. Acute postoperative pain. In: Miller RD (ed.), *Anaesthesia*. Edinburgh: Churchill Livingstone, 1994, pp. 2327–44.

Thomas TA, Griffiths MJ. A pain slide rule. *Anaesthesia* 1982; **37**:960–1.

Welchew EA. A postoperative pain recorder: a patient-controlled device for assessing postoperative pain. *Anaesthesia* 1982; **37**:838–41.

2 Patient-controlled analgesia (PCA)

> What are the advantages and disadvantages of intravenous patient-controlled analgesia for postoperative pain control?

Patient-controlled analgesia has a range of well-documented advantages compared with conventional analgesia. The regimen most commonly compared with intravenous PCA is the intramuscular 'as necessary' regimen.

Advantages and disadvantages

Advantages

1. There is consistently high patient satisfaction.
2. It provides equal or superior analgesia compared with other regimens.
3. There is equivalent or reduced sedation.
4. There is minimal delay in the onset of pain relief.
5. There is individual tailoring of analgesia to the patient's needs.
6. The patient retains a sense of being 'in control'.
7. There is some evidence for shorter hospital stays.
8. There is some evidence for fewer pulmonary complications.

Disadvantages

1. The cost is increased.
2. There is possible overdose due to machine-related or human failure.
3. Patient education is required.
4. Nurse education is required (diversity of types of pump).
5. There is a necessity for an acute pain team.
6. It is not useful for spasmodic pain.
7. It delivers small bolus doses.
8. Demands are initiated by pain.

Discussion

A well-run conventional analgesic regimen can provide good-quality analgesia compared with intravenous PCA. The problem is that we know that conventional regimens do not seem to be well administered because of poor ward design, depleted nursing levels and inadequate training.

The principal advantage of PCA is that the patient's pain should be reduced to tolerable levels. Respiratory depression does not appear to be a problem except when buprenorphine is used, despite a wide range in the number of demands and total amount of drug delivered.

The disadvantages are many. When the pain is spasmodic, the method is unlikely to be helpful and may lead to toxicity. Because the individual doses are small, analgesia may require many demands over a significant period. Since the demands are initiated by pain, some pain is likely to be present for most of the time. If the drug is rapid in its onset and offset, the frequency of demand is high. During confusion or sleep demands will not be made despite the consequences of noxious stimuli in terms of vasoconstriction, truncated breathing etc.

Further reading

Farmer M, Harper NJ. Unexpected problems with patient controlled analgesia. *Br Med J* 1992; **304**:574.

Finley RJ, Keeri-Szanto M. New analgesic agents and techniques shorten post-operative hospital stay. *Pain* 1982; **3**(suppl.):S397.

Gibbs JM, Johnson HD, Davis FM. Patient administration of IV buprenorphine for postoperative pain relief using the 'Cardiff' demand analgesia apparatus. *Br J Anaesth* 1982; **54**:279–84.

Ross EL, Pemmberti P. PCA: is it cost effective when used for postoperative pain management? *Anaesthesiology* 1988; **69**:A710.

Scalley RD, Berquist K, Cochran RS. Patient controlled analgesia in orthopaedic procedures. *Orthop Rev* 1988; **17**:1106–13.

Wasylak TJ, Abbott FV, English MJM, Jeans ME. Reduction of postoperative morbidity following patient controlled analgesia. *Can J Anaesth* 1990; **37**:726–31.

Welchew EA. On-demand analgesia: a double-blind comparison of on-demand intravenous fentanyl with regular intramuscular morphine. *Anaesthesia* 1983; **38**:19–25.

3   Safety of PCA

What safety features should be incorporated into a patient-controlled analgesia (PCA) system and what is the purpose of each? What instructions would you give to the nursing staff, having set up the PCA?

In 1976 the first commercially available device for providing patient-controlled analgesia was described by Evans and colleagues. This device was easy to tamper with, cumbersome and simple but reliable. Developments in PCA since that time have resulted in reduced size, lighter weight, tamperproofing, robustness, stepper motors, digital pulses, microprocessors, memory and programs to control infusions. However, several cases of overdose have been reported with PCA.

The main safety features of a PCA system include:

- lockable pumps
- protocols
- patient-safe mode when deprogrammed
- pre-filled syringes
- siphoning effects
- standard prescriptions
- phantom hand
- locking clamp.

Discussion

One of the keys to solving programming errors is to have one model of pump on a single site and use uniform programs on all of the machines. This simple program can be used with children as long as the opiate-containing syringes are customised to the weight of the child.

The syringes should be locked into the PCA pumps and the keys to the locks should themselves be locked in the drugs cupboard with a copy of the pump protocol.

Written protocols with clear instructions for setting up the pumps should be established and available whenever the pumps are set up. A clear written protocol for refilling the pumps should also be available on every ward using them. Only trained personnel should be allowed to set up or refill the pumps.

Many pumps will lose their program settings if their power supply is interrupted. When the power is restored staff may be unaware that the pump has lost its program settings. Several pumps currently available may be deprogrammed by static electricity. Anti-static sprays applied to the extension of the pumps may prevent this. The only safeguard is to use machines that stop in a patient-safe mode when deprogrammed.

Pre-filled syringes containing the standard opiate dilution prepared in an aseptic environment should be available 24 hours a day from the pharmacy. If, however, different drugs or dilutes are used in the same syringes it is possible for staff to mix them up. This may occur when concentrations of opiate are calculated on a weight basis for children, when syringes of the same size are used for analgesics given by other routes (e.g. epidural), when drugs with similar sounding names but different potencies are used in the same hospital (e.g. morphine and diamorphine), or if pharmacy supplies a range of other drugs such as insulin or heparin in similar syringes.

At least two cases have been reported of accidental siphoning of opiate out of the syringe and into the patient, leading to an overdose. This can occur only if there is a sufficiently high hydrostatic pressure in the liquid of the syringe to force it under its own weight down the tubing into the patient. If the syringe is 30 cm or more above the cannula in the patient then siphoning may occur. Thus pumps must always be fixed at the same height as the cannula in the patient so that the effective hydrostatic pressure is zero, and all giving sets should include an anti-siphon valve to prevent air getting into the syringe from the giving set with a sufficiently high resistance to flow to stop liquid moving because of hydrostatic pressure.

To avoid prescription errors, a 'standard prescription' should be used throughout the hospital. All adults should have the same prescription and all children the same prescription formula. Any variation from the standard prescription must be discussed with the acute pain team. Although there are great advantages to this system, the disadvantage is that variations in sensitivity to the bolus dose are not taken into account. Faulty prescriptions when using this system become rare if, additionally, different coloured stickers for the drug prescription charts, or different charts altogether, are used for intravenous, epidural or paediatric prescriptions.

The bolus button should be pressed only by the patient to maintain the operant conditioning loop which causes the frequency of button pressing to be related to the magnitude of pain. If this loop is broken there is a potential for overdose. All members of staff on wards using PCA machines must be thoroughly warned of the danger of allowing anyone other than the patient to press the button.

Patients or their relatives may attempt to reprogram the PCA machine to give more analgesic, or attempt to remove the entire PCA machine in order to obtain the enclosed opiate. Machines should always have a locking clamp to fix them to the patient's bed.

Further reading

Evans UM, MacCarthy J, Rosen M, Hogg MIJ. Apparatus for patient controlled administration of narcotics during labour. *Lancet* 1976; **i**:M-8.

Harmer M, Rosen M, Vickers MD (eds). *Patient Controlled Analgesia*. Oxford: Blackwell Scientific, 1984, pp. 57–72.

Lam FY. Patient controlled analgesia by proxy. *Br J Anaesth* 1993; **70**:113.

Rowbotham DJ. The development and safe use of patient-controlled analgesia. *Br J Anaesth* 1992; **68**:331–2 (editorial).

Stevens DS, Cohen RI, Kanzaria RV, Dunn WT. Air in the syringe: patient controlled analgesia machine tampering. *Anaesthesiology* 1991; **75**:697–9.

White PF. Mishaps with patient controlled analgesia. *Anaesthesiology* 1987; **66**:81–83.

4 NSAIDs

> What are the indications for the use of non-steroidal anti-inflammatory drugs (NSAIDs) in current anaesthetic practice? Give details of their administration, modes of action and side-effects.

The non-steroidal anti-inflammatory drugs are probably the most widely used group of drugs in the world. Indications for their use are:
- acute pain following surgery
- renal colic
- chronic pain arising from inflammation
- opioid-sparing
- prophylactic treatment of cardiovascular and thrombotic related diseases
- antipyretic effect.

Administration

1. PR (rectal).
2. IM (intramuscular).
3. IV (intravenous).
4. Oral.

Side-effects

1. Gastric toxicity.
2. Renal complications.
3. Haemostatic impairment.
4. CNS toxicity.
5. Dermatological effects.
6. Aspirin-induced asthma.
7. Haematological effects.
8. Hepatotoxicity.
9. Teratogenic effects.
10. Drug interactions.

Discussion

NSAIDs are being used increasingly in the early postoperative phase after minor and superficial operations and in the later postoperative phase after major operations. NSAIDs alone are insufficient to provide postoperative analgesia after major surgery.

There is no evidence that pre-emptive analgesia occurs with NSAIDs, but when given in addition to opioids they have been shown to have an opioid-sparing effect. Studies combining the use of NSAIDs with bupivacaine–

morphine epidurals have not shown any improvement in analgesia and mobilisation. Studies in patients after major abdominal and thoracic surgery have shown that NSAIDs given soon after operations reduce opioid requirement by about one-third in the first two postoperative days. This has been shown with intramuscular ketorolac, rectal indomethacin and rectal ibuprofen.

NSAIDs provide potent and rapid analgesia for patients suffering with renal colic. Often the entire episode of renal colic can be covered by a single dose of a non-steroidal.

There has been increased interest in the postoperative use of NSAIDs as analgesics in children. The incidence of unwanted side-effects in children is low. There is little data to determine the dose recommendations in children, however.

Aspirin and other NSAIDs are being increasingly used to prevent cardiovascular and thrombotic disease. The beneficial effects of the drugs relate to their ability to block platelet cyclo-oxygenase activity and hence stop platelet aggregation. Aspirin irreversibly acetylates platelet cyclo-oxygenase and once destroyed it is not replaced, the effect lasting for the lifetime of the platelet (7–10 days). Most of the other NSAIDs reversibly inhibit cyclo-oxygenase enzyme activity, returning on removal of the drug.

NSAIDs must be given carefully to patients already on anticoagulant therapy. Aspirin may be associated with increased postoperative bleeding. If there is considered to be a risk of bleeding, treatment should be changed to paracetamol or a short-acting non-steroidal such as ibuprofen or ketoprofen, which can be stopped prior to surgery.

Diclofenac, a phenylacetic acid derivative possessing analgesic, anti-inflammatory and antipyretic activity, is widely used in the UK. It can be given orally, by deep intramuscular injection or as a suppository. The maximum dose by any route is 150mg per day. Absorption of NSAIDs from the gastrointestinal tract is usually excellent and for most NSAIDs bioavailability is nearly 100%. Diclofenac is an exception in so far as it undergoes extensive first-pass hepatic metabolism such that only 50% of the drug is available systemically following oral ingestion. Diclofenac is available for use in children one year of age or over, the maximum dose being 3mg/kg per day in divided doses.

NSAIDs inhibit cyclo-oxygenase, blocking the pathway leading to the formation of prostaglandins. All nucleated cells synthesise prostaglandins when the cell membrane is damaged. This leads to the production of prostaglandin, prostacyclin and thromboxane. Some of these substances stimulate nociceptive nerve endings directly; others sensitise the nerve endings to further stimulation. The normally high-threshold nociceptors fire more frequently in response to normal stimulation, leading to an increase in sensitivity to pain in the area surrounding the trauma.

One of the major side-effects of non-steroidals is upper gastrointestinal ulceration and bleeding. Dyspepsia is the most common adverse effect, occurring in about 10% of subjects treated with newer non-steroidals. There is inter-patient variability in the occurrence of dyspepsia with different NSAIDS. The relationship between dyspepsia and upper GI damage is not clear. Of great importance is the risk of major bleeding or perforation of peptic ulcers by NSAIDs. Males and females over 60 years of age admitted to hospital with bleeding duodenal or gastric ulcers are three to four times more likely to be taking NSAIDs than the matched controls. Reducing the dosage, the use of enteric-coated forms of drugs, taking the drugs on a prn basis, the avoidance of the long-half-life NSAIDs in the elderly and of combinations of NSAIDs which potentiate gastrointestinal damage, can all decrease gastric toxicity.

The incidence of renal toxicity with NSAIDs use is low. There is increased incidence of renal dysfunction in advanced age, cirrhosis of the liver, dehydration, congestive cardiac failure, gastrointestinal haemorrhage and pre-existing renal disease.

The most common renal condition associated with NSAIDs is acute renal failure that is ischaemic in origin. It is usually reversible if NSAIDs are stopped but can be severe enough to cause tubular necrosis. Acute renal failure usually occurs within 24 hours of commencing treatment and may occur after one dose. It is particularly likely to occur in dehydrated subjects, and in anyone suffering from systemic lupus erythematosus, chronic glomerulonephritis, and cirrhosis of the liver with ascites or heart failure. In certain circumstances prostaglandin I_2 produced locally in the renal cortex and the medulla is required to maintain renal perfusion in the face of vasoconstrictive influences, such as angiotensin II, antidiuretic hormone and catecholamines. A number of cases of acute renal failure have been reported following administration of almost all of the available NSAIDs.

The development of acute tubulointerstitial nephritis and the nephritic syndrome can occur with NSAID therapy. This syndrome can develop within weeks or after years of NSAID treatment. An underlying renal disease does not appear to be a risk factor; the mechanism appears to be allergic in nature due to T-lymphocyte activation. It is impossible to predict who will develop nephritis but it is usually seen in older patients.

All NSAIDs can produce renal papillary necrosis. Prostaglandin synthesis inhibition and hence medullary ischaemia, may be responsible for, or contribute to, renal papillary necrosis. Chronic renal failure associated with NSAIDs is unlike classical analgesic-induced nephropathy as it is seen most commonly in the elderly and in men and not in women of 30–40 years of age.

NSAIDs have been shown to cause central nervous system side-effects. Up to 10% of patients taking NSAIDs suffer effects of varying severity, such as headache, depression and tinnitus. This adverse effect may be due to direct action on blood vessels.

The most common dermatological reactions of the NSAIDs are erythematous macular rashes and pruritus, which resolve on cessation of the drug. On very rare occasions, the use of any of the non-steroidals may cause severe idiosyncratic skin reactions, such as erythema multiforme, pemphigus vulgaris or exfoliative dermatitis.

Asthmatics have a 4–20% chance of developing an asthmatic attack precipitated by aspirin or other NSAIDs. The clinical picture of NSAID intolerance is very characteristic. The first symptoms appear during the years 20–40. The disease starts with malaise, nasal discharge, coughing and sneezing. These symptoms resolve within a week or two. Rhinitis persists, however, and polyps develop. The combination of asthma, aspirin intolerance and nasal polyps has been described as the aspirin triad. Within 1 hour following ingestion of aspirin, acute asthma develops with rhinorrhoea, conjunctiva irritation and scarlet flush of the head and neck. These attacks range from asthma to severe anaphylactoid reaction. This serious effect of aspirin is not a classic type I allergic response. It appears to be related to cyclo-oxygenase inhibition. There is a 10% cross-reaction rate with paracetamol – increasing the dose increases the chance of a reaction.

Hepatic toxicity can occur with all the NSAIDs. It ranges from a mild elevation of transaminases to fulminant liver failure and death. Treatment with an NSAID should be discontinued if there is any indication of more severe hepatotoxicity, such as prolonged prothrombin time. The most common hepatotoxic adverse effect of NSAIDs is a transient asymptomatic elevation of plasma transaminases.

Further reading

Carmichael J, Shankel SW. Effects of nonsteroidal anti-inflammatory drugs on prostaglandins and renal function. *Am J Med* 1985; **78**:992.

Crossley RJ. Side effect and safety data for fenbufen. *Am J Med* 1983; **75**:84–90.

Gilles GWA, Kenny GNC, Bullingham RES, McArdle CS. Morphine-sparing effect of ketoralic tromerhamine, a new parenteral non-steroidal anti-inflammatory agent, following abdominal surgery. *Anaesthesia* 1987; **42**:727–31.

Magrini M, Pavesi G, Liverta C, Bruni G. Intravenous ketoprofen in renal colic: a placebo-controlled pilot study. *Clin Ther* 1984; **6**:483–7.

Mogensen T, Vegger P, Johnsson T *et al*. Systemic piroxicam as an adjunct to combined epidural bupivacaine and morphine for postoperative pain relief- a double blind study. *Anaesth Analg* 1992; **74**:363–70.

Snyder RD, Siegal GL. An asthma trial. *Ann Allergy* 1967; **25**:377.

Somerville K, Faulkner G, Langham M. Non-steroidal anti-inflammatory drugs and bleeding peptic ulcer. *Lancet* 1986; **i**: 462–4.

5 Complex regional pain syndrome

> A 60-year-old man is referred with reflex sympathetic dystrophy following an injury at the elbow six months earlier. Outline the treatment.

Complex regional pain syndrome type I (CRPS I) was formerly known as 'reflex sympathetic dystrophy' or Sudeck's atrophy.

Diagnosis

Accurate diagnosis of the CRPS is important as early diagnosis and treatment may improve outcome. For a diagnosis of CRPS I, the following two criteria must be present:

- continuing pain, allodynia or hyperalgesia which is disproportionate to the inciting event
- evidence at some time of oedema, changes in blood flow or abnormal sudomotor activity in the region of the pain.

Diagnosis is excluded by the existence of conditions that would otherwise account for the degree of pain and dysfunction.

There does not have to be an initiating noxious event or cause of immobilisation to make the diagnosis of CRPS I.

Pain is localised to the limb and described as deep and burning. The limb is painful to move and demonstrates allodynia and hyperalgesia. It is swollen and often shiny. There may be trophic changes in nails and loss of hair; the affected limb may be abnormally warm or abnormally cool.

The diagnosis of CRPS is a clinical one. History and examination findings are reinforced by the x-ray findings of localised osteoporosis, but a diagnosis can be made without x-ray findings. Early recognition of the condition and aggressive treatment is important with regard to outcome.

Management

Management strategies are:

- intravenous or regional neural sympathetic blocks
- drug therapy
- psychosocial support
- spinal cord stimulation
- free radical scavengers.

Relief provided by intravenous phentolamine (0.5–1 mg/kg infused over 20 minutes) suggests that the pain is likely to respond to *sympathetic blockade* which can be performed by intravenous or regional neural sympathetic blocks. Classically, intravenous sympathetic blockade is performed by the injection of guanethidine into a limb isolated with a tourniquet.

Although there is no scientific evidence to support intravenous regional sympathetic blockade, anecdotal evidence is strong and the technique is often practised. Other drugs such as bretylium, ketanserin, droperidol and reserpine have been used for intravenous regional sympathetic blockade, with only ketanserin showing any benefit. Systemic sympathetic blockade can be obtained from drugs such as clonidine, guanethidine or beta-blockers.

Maintenance of mobility is central to improvement of CRPS and prevention of secondary features. If pain is relieved by sympathetic nervous system blockade, a block can be used to give a period of analgesia during which physiotherapy can be intensive.

Antidepressants, anticonvulsants and other membrane stabilisers, which are used to treat other neuropathic pains, offer therapeutic possibilities. *Psychological support* is important to minimise disability, which results from behavioural changes. *Spinal cord stimulation* relieved pain and reduced swelling in a small series of patients. Recent work suggests a role for *free radical scavengers* such as mannitol.

Further reading

Charlton JE. Reflex sympathetic dystrophy: non-invasive methods of treatment. In: Stanton-Hicks M, Janig W, Boas RA (eds), *Reflex Sympathetic Dystrophy*. Boston: Kluwer, 1990, pp. 151–64.

Jadad AR, Carroll D, Glynn CJ, McQuay HJ. Intravenous regional sympathetic blockade for pain relief in reflex sympathetic dystrophy: a systemic review and a randomised double-blind crossover study. *J Pain Sympt Manag* 1995; **10**:13–20.

Jang W, Stanton-Hicks H (eds). *Reflex Sympathetic Dystrophy: a Reappraisal*. Seattle: IASP Press, 1989.

Paice E. Fortnightly review: reflex sympathetic dystrophy. *Br Med J* 1995; **310**:164–7.

6 Neurogenic pain

List (with examples) the causes of neurogenic pain. What symptoms are produced? What treatments are available?

Causes

Neurogenic or neuropathic pain is associated with abnormality, injury or disease in the nervous system. This includes:
- painful mononeuropathies (e.g. intercostal neuralgia)
- polyneuropathies (e.g. diabetes mellitus)
- deafferentation pain (e.g. brachial plexus avulsion, central post-stroke pain)
- systemically maintained pain (may or may not be associated with nerve injury)
- scar pain
- post-herpetic neuralgia
- spinal cord injury
- complex regional pain syndromes.

Symptoms

Nerve damage at any point of the sensory system may result in any of the following features:
- spontaneous pain which may be paroxysmal
- pain described as burning, shooting or numb
- severe pain in response to a noxious stimulus (hyperalgesia)
- severe pain in response to a stimulus which is not normally noxious (allodynia)
- severe pain in response to stimulation despite sensory impairment (hyperpathia).

Similar clinical entities may produce different symptoms in different patients.

Principles of management

Many treatment methods for chronic pain enjoy a brief vogue before fading from use because they ignore the multidimensional nature of the problem. No two pains are the same and individualisation of management, usually with a combination of therapies, produces the best results. The principles of management of neurogenic pain can be listed as:
- prevention
- remove cause
- medication
- neural blockade
- stimulation-induced analgesia

- neurosurgery
- physical therapy
- psychology.

Optimal *perioperative analgesia* might prevent chronic postsurgical pain. Sympathetic blocks may reduce the incidence of post-herpetic neuralgesia during the acute zoster stage. The incidence of phantom limb pain may be reduced by epidural analgesia 48 hours prior to lower-limb amputation, although recent work contradicts this treatment.

Surgery, radiotherapy or medication may modify the pathophysiological process leading to neurogenic pain.

NSAIDs and related drugs are indicated when there is ongoing peripheral tissue damage. In patients with opioid-sensitive pain there is evidence that the long-term use of *opioids* is safe and the psychological dependence is almost never observed. *Antidepressants*, particularly non-selective ones such as amitriptyline, are effective for neuropathic pain, central stroke pain, atypical facial pain and fibromyalgia. The analgesic effect is separate from the antidepressant effect and occurs at lower doses. *Anticonvulsants*, particularly carbamazepine, are useful for trigeminal neuralgia, diabetic neuropathy and other conditions with lightning or shooting pains. *Membrane-stabilising drugs* such as mexiletine can be used for neuropathic pain. *Adrenergic blocks*, such as with phenoxybenzamine, as well as *corticosteroids* and many other drugs, have been recommended for sympathetically maintained pain. Guanethidine or bretylium can be used in an intravenous regional technique. Painful spasms associated with spinal cord injury or multiple sclerosis may respond to baclofen or dantrolene.

Peripheral nerve blocks are indicated for pains such as ilioinguinal neuralgia and neuralgia paraesthetica. Epidural and facet joint injections are employed for lower back pain. Chemical sympathectomy is a very effective treatment for rest pain and skin ulceration due to occlusive vascular disease. Local anaesthetic sympathetic blocks or intravenous regional blocks are used for complex regional pain syndrome (reflex sympathetic dystrophy). Coeliac plexus block may relieve the pain of chronic pancreatitis. The substances injected include local anaesthetic steroids, neurolytic solutions such as phenol or alcohol.

Physical methods use cryolesions or radio-frequency thermocoagulation. The clinical response to acupuncture and TENS is variable and unpredictable but some patients do gain significant benefit. Acupuncture may produce changes in spinal cord neurotransmitter concentrations. Transcutaneous electrical nerve stimulation (TENS) is derived from the gate theory of pain. Headaches, musculoskeletal disorders and some neuropathic pains may respond well to these techniques. Implanted peripheral nerve stimulation has been used for some neuropathic pains. Spinal cord stimulation offers relief to a limited group of patients; suggested indications include arachnoiditis, peripheral vascular disease and intractable angina.

Exercise and strengthening exercises are of more benefit than rest and 'back schools' reinforce these concepts. Manipulation may be useful for acute episodes of back pain but is of less benefit in chronic cases. Rehabilitation programmes can be vital even for cases with irreversible damage such as avulsion lesions of the brachial plexus. Physical therapies include exercise therapy, orthotics, manipulation, ultrasound, back school and rehabilitation programmes.

Enthusiasm for *neurosurgical intervention* has waned considerably in recent years with the realisation that cutting the nervous system anywhere is rarely the answer to chronic pain. Dorsal root entry zone (DREZ) lesioning is indicated in deafferentation pain following brachial plexus avulsion. Vascular decompression of the trigeminal nerve relieves some cases of trigeminal neuralgia.

Psychological and behavioural approaches to chronic pain management are useful for many patients, but participation of the spouse or family is vital. Cognitive–behavioural programmes are indicated for patients for whom there is no effective treatment. The aim is to achieve the best possible level of physical and emotional function within the confines of the condition. Pain reduction is not the aim but may follow the improvement in function. Psychological approaches to chronic pain management include education, self-monitoring, relaxation, desensitisation, coping strategies, cognitive therapy, anxiety management, psychotherapy and biofeedback.

Further reading

Bowsher D. Neurogenic pain syndromes and their management. *Br Med Bull* 1991; **47**:644–66.

Charlton JE. Reflex sympathetic dystrophy: non-invasive methods of treatment. In: Stanton-Hicks M, Janig W, Baas RA (eds), *Reflex Sympathetic Dystrophy*. Boston: Kluwer, 1990, pp. 151–64.

Flor H, Fydrich T, Turk DC. Efficacy of multi-discipinary pain treatment centres: a meta analytic review. *Pain* 1992; **49**:221–30.

Melzack R, Wall PD. Pain mechanisms: a new theory. *Science* 1965; **150**:971–9.

Merskey H for the International Association for the Study of Pain. Classification of chronic pain: descriptions of chronic syndromes and definitions of pain terms. *Pain* 1986; suppl. 3.

7 Stellate ganglion block

> **What are the indications for, and complications of, stellate ganglion block?**

The inferior cervical sympathetic ganglion is fused with the first thoracic ganglion in about 80% of subjects; this combined structure is termed the stellate ganglion.

In order to obtain therapeutic effect, a series of blocks is usually required – e.g. one block each day over a period of 4–5 days. Stellate ganglion block should be combined with other conventional forms of treatment such as physiotherapy, protection from cold etc.

Indications

The indications are:

- regional circulatory insufficiency:
  - Raynaud's disease
  - arterial embolism
  - post-traumatic syndrome
- sympathetically maintained pain
- severe angina pectoris
- complex regional pain syndrome.

Complications

Complications of stellate ganglion block are:

- haematoma
- recurrent laryngeal nerve paralysis or partial involvement of the brachial plexus
- intravascular injection
- dural puncture
- osteitis
- mediastinitis.

Haematoma occurs fairly readily and hampers subsequent blocks but usually requires no treatment. Intravascular injection of an appreciable amount of local anaesthetic solution, especially into the vertebral artery, should be prevented by repeated aspiration. The injection should always be administered slowly, the patient being watched carefully for any sign of toxic reaction to the local anaesthetic agent – such as dizziness or unconsciousness.

Dural puncture cannot normally be diagnosed by the spontaneous back-flow of cerebrospinal fluid, or by aspiration, because the hydrostatic pressure in the dural cuffs protruding through the intervertebral foramina is low. The dura itself is very thin in this area and may easily occlude the aperture of the needle. Subarachnoid injection would result in widespread spinal anaesthesia, commencing in the cervical region, where it would be most intense.

Osteitis in the transverse process is a rare complication and may be caused by oesophageal perforation by the needle prior to approaching the transverse process.

Mediastinitis with formation of intrathoracic abscess has been described.

Further reading

Prithvi Raj P, Anderson SR. In: Waldman SD (ed.), *Interventional Pain Management*, 2nd edn. Philadelphia: WB Saunders.

8 Postoperative pain

A 60-year-old man presents for a hemicolectomy. How may choice of pain management influence recovery from surgery?

The choices for managing acute pain following hemicolectomy are diverse. Analgesic drugs which have an effect postoperatively may be given in the preoperative, perioperative or postoperative periods. No single route or technique is able to produce zero pain scores and a combined approach is often required.

Postoperative pain causes patient discomfort and distress, hyperventilation and respiratory alkalosis, increased oxygen demand and metabolic acidosis, an increased neuroendocrine stress response, reduced immunological function, delayed postoperative mobilisation and an increased risk of deep vein thrombosis (DVT).

Routes of administration

These are:
* intramuscular
* intravenous
* subcutaneous
* rectal
* local anaesthetic infiltration or nerve blocks
* epidural and subarachnoid block
* oral.

Discussion

Opioid analgesics are frequently given intramuscularly but analgesia is slow owing to the slow development of peak systemic concentrations. The level of the peak concentration is likely to be lower than that following intravenous administration. Injections are painful and dosage is fixed so that it may be too small or too large. The time interval between doses may permit breakthrough pain, and pain control is removed from the sufferer.

Intermittent intravenous bolus doses of opioid analgesics are usually administered by anaesthetic staff or nursing staff in high-dependency areas. Systemic levels of the drug may fluctuate rapidly and there is a risk of serious side-effects including respiratory depression. Systemic side-effects are rarely a problem if the drug is titrated against analgesic effect.

Large interpersonal variations in drug requirements are largely overcome with the use of patient-controlled analgesia (PCA). Using PCA patients are able to take responsibility for the balance between acceptable levels of pain and acceptable levels of side-effects from analgesic agents. There is no means of predicting the minimum effective analgesic concentration (MEAC) in an individual, so patients using PCA are able to maintain a relatively constant drug level around their individual MEAC level.

Subcutaneous injections or infusions of opioids are an alternative route to the intramuscular route. The subcutaneous route is more frequently used in children than adults since small cannulae can be inserted with minimal distress, or in adults who are very thin with little muscle bulk.

The rectal route is not as popular in the UK as in other countries. Systemic absorption avoids first-pass elimination. It is not affected by gastrointestinal motility or postoperative nausea and vomiting (PONV), but slow absorption delays onset – non-steroidal anti-inflammatory drugs (NSAIDs) are often administered rectally to great effect.

Local anaesthetic techniques have the advantage of complete avoidance of the side-effects of opioids. Nerve blocks which are functioning prior to surgery may abolish the stress response. For the pain caused by a laparotomy for hemicolectomy, bilateral intercostal nerve blocks or interpleural catheters may not provide adequate postoperative analgesia as the intercostal nerve blocks may require a top-up and hence be repeated; they do not block visceral pain fibres; and there is a significant risk of pneumothorax using this technique. Local infiltration of the wound or intercostal nerve may be used successfully in conjunction with opioids delivered by various routes.

Further reading

Postoperative pain relief: what is the issue? *Br J Anaesth* 1994; **72**:375–7 (editorial).

Kuhn S, Cooke S, Collins M, Jones LM, Mucklow JC. Perceptions on pain relief after surgery. *Br Med J* 1990; **300**:1687–90.

Royal College of Surgeons of England, and College of Anaesthetists. *Commission on the Provision of Surgical Services: Report of the Working Party on Pain after Surgery*. London: HMSO, 1990.

9 The postanaesthetic visit

> What information would you wish to obtain from a patient at your postanaesthetic visit, the day after a total hip replacement?

The postanaesthetic visit 24 hours after total hip replacement should encompass a clinical assessment of the patient as well as a review of laboratory investigations and the drug prescription chart.

Patients presenting for total hip replacement are often elderly and have coexisting diseases with increased risk of deep vein thrombosis (DVT) and pulmonary embolus, increased risk of pneumonia and, thus, increased overall mortality.

Clinical assessment

This should consist of:
* pain management
* PONV (postoperative nausea and vomiting)
* systemic assessment of cardiovascular and respiratory systems
* urine output and hydration status
* cognitive function
* DVT
* pressure areas
* neurological assessment.

Clinical assessment of the patient should include examining for evidence of deep vein thrombosis. Orthopaedic patients represent the highest risk group for DVT, with 45–70% incidence in those undergoing hip or knee reconstructive surgery. Prolonged surgery is an added risk factor. Specific therapy to prevent DVT is heparin 5000 IU t.d.s. or low-molecular-weight heparin (shown to halve the incidence of DVT in surgical patients). Graduated compression stockings have been shown to halve the incidence, as have intermittent pneumatic compression boots used preoperatively and for 16 hours postoperatively.

Following total hip replacement, patients should have a full blood count, as 10–20% of blood volume will extravasate around the prosthesis in the immediate postoperative period.

Laboratory investigations

To include:
* full blood count (FBC)
* urea and electrolytes
* ECG as necessary
* clotting as necessary.

Review of drug prescription chart

To include:

* normal regular medication
* prophylactic antibiotics
* DVT prophylactics.

Discussion

Postoperative pain management depends on which technique of acute pain management has been used. Regional anaesthetic techniques (spinal or epidural) are commonly used in major orthopaedic lower-limb procedures because of better earlier postoperative gas exchange, reduced blood transfusion requirements, reduced bleeding from the bone, improved cardiovascular stability, improved postoperative mental function, reduced incidence of DVT, and good postoperative analgesia.

Postanaesthesia hypotension may occur if a continuous epidural infusion is used.

In the elderly, occlusion of intervertebral foramina results in a more variable and usually smaller dose requirement. Both the total amount of local anaesthetic drug and concentration of drug determine the level of motor block. Epidural and spinal opioids decrease local anaesthetic requirements and so reduce motor blockade and improve pain relief. Increasing lipophilicity results in greater systemic action of opioids. The low lipophilicity of morphine results in rostral migration of drug in the cerebrospinal fluid (CSF) and may cause delayed respiratory depression. There may be respiratory impairment if the block is too high, causing impaired force of cough and bronchoconstriction.

Headache following spinal anaesthesia or dural tap during an epidural may be due to dural stretching caused by the weight of the brain above the tentorium transmitted via the trigeminal nerve to the frontal region. It is most common in young fit patients and least common in the elderly. Spinal haematoma presents as a sudden onset of sharp backache and sciatica and occurs in approximately 1 in 50 000 epidural blocks. The incidence has increased since the introduction of low-molecular-weight heparin.

Other complications of regional anaesthesia are spinal abscess (presents with fever and back pain over 1–3 days), urinary retention and gastrointestinal effects due to loss of sympathetic inhibition resulting in small bowel contraction.

The incidence of PONV following epidural morphine is 20%. Central opioids commonly cause pruritus with an incidence of 46% following intrathecal administration and 8.5% after epidural administration. This can be treated with naloxone (5–10 μg/kg/h), propofol (10 mg) or droperidol (2.5 mg). The incidence of respiratory depression is 0.09% with extradural morphine and

0.36% following spinal morphine and can occur up to 24 hours after administration. It is more common if the patient is supine, following rapid intrathecal injection, in the elderly, in the presence of increased intra-abdominal pressure, with other respiratory depressants and with respiratory disease.

PONV in adults decreases with age and may be increased by preoperative anxiety due to catecholamine-induced delayed gastric emptying or a central emetogenic effect. Adult females are 2–4 times more likely to experience PONV, which is further increased if the patient receives opioids. Similarly, a previous history of PONV increases the likelihood of future PONV significantly. Opioids should be avoided in the postoperative period if possible and use should be made of NSAIDs (non-steroidal anti-inflammatory drugs). Avoid sudden movement and changes in posture, which may aggravate PONV. Early intake of food should be discouraged. If the patient experiences emesis, attention should be paid to hydration and pain management. If one antiemetic is unsuccessful, a drug with a different mechanism of action should be tried.

Further reading

Berquist D, Lindblad B, MatzschT. Low molecular weight herapin for thromboprophylaxis and epidural/spinal anaesthesia: is there a risk? *Acta Anaesth Scand* 1992; **36**:605–9.

Colditz G *et al*. Rates of venous thrombosis after general surgery: combined results of randomised clinical trials. *Lancet* 1986; **2**:143–6.

Covert CR, Fox GS. Anaesthesia for hip surgery in the elderly. *Can J Anaesth* 1989; **36**:311–19.

Davis M. Anaesthesia for major orthopaedic surgery in the elderly. *Curr Anaesth Crit Care* 1992; **3**:193–9.

Mason A, Palazzo M. *Postoperative Nausea and Vomiting*. New York: Churchill Livingstone, 1999.

Wildsmith JAW. Extradural abscess after central neural blockade. *Br J Anaesth* 1993; **70**:387–8.

Yeager MP, Glass DD, Neff RK, Brinck-Johnsen T. Epidural anaesthesia and analgesia in high-risk surgical patients. *Anaesthesiology* 1987; **66**:729–36.

Multiple-choice questions: Pain management

1. Intravenous guanethidine:
   a) blocks parasympathetic nerves
   b) cannot be repeated
   c) when used for the treatment of chronic pain the tourniquet must remain inflated for at least 1 hour
   d) is used as a treatment for sympathetic dystrophy
   e) commonly causes postural hypotension.

2. Trigeminal ganglion block causes ipsilateral analgesia of the:
   a) lower lip
   b) alar nasi
   c) angle of the jaw
   d) external auditory meatus
   e) soft palate.

3. Sympathetic dystrophy:
   a) can cause osteoporosis
   b) causes an increase in skin temperature
   c) causes pain
   d) causes vasoconstriction
   e) is more common in athletes.

4. Coeliac plexus blockade:
   a) can be used to relieve pain from intra-abdominal malignancy
   b) may cause orthostatic hypotension
   c) may cause diarrhoea
   d) can be used to treat pain in acute pancreatitis
   e) causes constriction of the sphincter of Oddi.

5. Complications of stellate ganglion block include:
   a) pneumothorax
   b) dural puncture
   c) injection into the vertebral artery
   d) damage to the phrenic nerve
   e) damage to the vagus nerve.

6. Sympathectomy may be used in the treatment of:
   a) Raynaud's disease
   b) causalgia
   c) hyperhydrosis
   d) venous ulcers
   e) pain of intermittent claudication.

7. Concerning stellate ganglion block:
   a) oesophageal perforation may occur
   b) diaphagmatic paralysis may result
   c) Horner's syndrome is essential for a successful block
   d) a successful block abolishes a change in skin resistance on stimulation
   e) a vasovagal reaction can occur whilst performing it.
8. The coeliac ganglion lies:
   a) on the body of the 13th vertebra
   b) in front of the aorta
   c) on the crura of the diaphragm
   d) behind the inferior vena cava
   e) behind the pancreas.

Answers to multiple-choice questions

1. a) False;   b) False;   c) False;   d) True;   e) False
2. a) True;   b) True;   c) False;   d) False;   e) False
3. a) False;   b) True;   c) True;   d) False;   e) False
4. a) True;   b) True;   c) True;   d) False;   e) False
5. a) True;   b) True;   c) True;   d) True;   e) True
6. a) True;   b) True;   c) True;   d) False;   e) True
7. a) True;   b) True;   c) True;   d) True;   e) True
8. a) False;   b) True;   c) True;   d) True;   e) True

1 Serum oxygen measurement

> Describe the physical principles that may be applied to the measurement of oxygen in the blood.

Measuring the tension, content or saturation of oxygen in the blood can assess oxygenation:
1. *Tension*
    - oxygen electrode
    - transcutaneous electrodes
    - fluorescence-based blood-gas analysis
    - ion-selective electrodes.
2. *Content and capacity*
    - volumetric method
    - blood haemolysis
    - galvanic cell
    - calorimetric method.
3. *Oxygen saturation*
    - oximetry.

Tension

The oxygen electrode (Clarke's electrode) consists of a platinum wire, normally 2 mm in diameter, which is embedded in a rough-surfaced glass rod. This is immersed in a phosphate buffer, which is stabilised with potassium chloride solution (KCl) and contained in an outer sachet. At the end of the outer jacket is a membrane, which is usually polyethylene or polypropylene, each being permeable to oxygen. The polyethylene membrane allows faster diffusion of oxygen than does polypropylene, making the system more sensitive but less stable. A polarising voltage of 600–800 mV is applied to the platinum wire and as oxygen diffuses through the membrane electro-oxidoreduction occurs at the cathode. Corresponding oxidation occurs at the Ag–AgCl anode. Thus a half-cell is set up and a current is generated.

The oxygen electrode in most blood gas analysers is calibrated using two standard gases, one containing no oxygen, the other about 12% O_2. Miniature electrodes have been used for the continuous intravascular monitoring of oxygen tension, but these are subject to a build-up of fibrin which alters the electrode sensitivity. The short response time of the electrode makes the system useful for monitoring acute changes in P_{O_2}.

Transcutaneous electrodes allow the monitoring of blood gases non-invasively, particularly when dealing with neonates and infants. The electrodes are based on similar principles to those used in blood gas analysers but also incorporate a heating element. The electrode is attached to the skin to form an airtight seal using a contact liquid, and the area is heated to 43°C. At this temperature the blood flow to the skin increases and the capillary oxygen diffuses through the skin, allowing measurement of the diffused gases by the attached electrode. Problems can occur with surgical diathermy where the heating current circuit provides a return path for the cutting current, causing the transcutaneous electrode to overheat. The values obtained from transcutaneous electrodes will generally be lower than those obtained from a simultaneous arterial specimen. The electrode reads low with severe hypertension and microcirculatory perfusion failure.

Fluorescence-based blood-gas analysis depends upon light from a pulsed xeron lamp being selectively filtered at 410, 460 and 385 nm for the respective measurement of pH, $P\text{CO}_2$ and $P\text{O}_2$. The $P\text{O}_2$ measurement utilises an oxygen-quenchable dye dissolved in silicone attached directly to the end of the sensor fibre. The dye is excited with light at 385 nm, and the decrease in light emitted at 515 nm is directly proportional to the oxygen tension. The sensor is coated in covalently bonded heparin, which is said to make it biocompatible for single use up to 72 hours.

The ion-selective or pH electrode utilises a glass membrane, the composition of which is tailored selectively to allow hydrogen ions to pass through, thus producing an electromotive force (EMF). The most commonly used electrode systems are those which are selective for sodium, potassium and calcium. The membranes, although different, all produce an electrical response when in contact with salt solution containing the particular ion to which the electrode is sensitive. The magnitude of the EMF is based on the Nernst equation. Systems incorporating ion-selective electrodes have the advantage that they can measure the relevant substances directly without the need for pretreatment or centrifuging. Minimal technique ability is required and they are virtually hazard-free.

Content and capacity

Various methods have been used to measure oxygen content and capacity. A volumetric method has been used whereby the gases dissolved in a blood sample were liberated using lactic acid and vacuum extraction and the volume measured at a fixed (atmospheric) pressure. This method is technically difficult and time-consuming and is now rarely used.

Another method of measuring O_2 content is to add a small sample of blood to a large volume (50 mL) of potassium ferricyanide solution. The latter haemolyses the red cells and drives the oxygen into solution. By measuring the $P\text{O}_2$ before and after adding the blood, and knowing the solubility of oxygen in the solution, it is possible to calculate the oxygen content of the original sample.

Oxygen content measurement is possible using a direct-reading galvanic cell system. Here a carrier gas consisting of 1% carbon monoxide, 2% hydrogen and 97% nitrogen is passed over a palladium catalyst (to ensure that it contains no oxygen) and bubbled through a haemolysed blood sample. The liberated oxygen is reduced at a carbon cathode, which gives rise to four electrons per molecule of oxygen. The current generated is proportional to the amount of oxygen in the sample. Although unaffected by the presence of volatile anaesthetic agents, this system is not widely used.

A calorimetric method of oxygen content measurement requires a 10-mL sample of whole blood to be injected anaerobically into a sealed cuvette containing an alkaline catachol solution, and the change in absorbency at 511 nm is measured. From this a blank representing fully reduced haemoglobin has to be subtracted, and this is obtained by injecting a similar volume of sample into an identical cuvette containing 0.1 molar sodium hydroxide.

Saturation

Oxygen saturation utilises the difference between the characteristic absorption spectra of haemoglobin and oxyhaemoglobin to quantify the relative concentrations of the two forms in the sample. It is discussed elsewhere in this section (see PULSE OXIMETRY).

Further reading

Clark LC. Monitoring and control of blood and tissue oxygen tension. *Trans Soc Artif Intern Organs* 1956; **2**:41–8.

Harabin AL, Farhi LE. Measurement of blood O_2 and CO_2 concentrations using Po_2 and Pco_2 electrodes. *J Appl Physiol* 1978; **44**:818–20.

Huch A, Huch R, Schneider H, Rooth G. Continuous transcutaneous monitoring of foetal oxygen during labour. *Br J Obstet Gynaecol* 1977; **84**(suppl. 1):1–39.

Miller WW, Masao Y, Cheng FY, Henry KH, Arick S. Performance of an in-vivo continuous blood-gas monitor with disposable probe. *Clin Chem* 1987; **33**:1538–42.

Selman BJ, White YS, Tait AR. An evaluation of the Sex-O_2-Con oxygen content analyser. *Anaesthesia* 1975; **30**:206–11.

Zander R, Lang W, Wolf HU. Oxygen cuvette: a simple approach to the oxygen concentration measurement in blood. *Pflugers Arch* 1977; **368**:R16.

2   Pulse oximetry

Describe the physical principles of pulse oximetry and indicate its limitations.

Principles

Spectrophotometric analysis of haemoglobin is based on the fact that if a mixture of oxyhaemoglobin and deoxyhaemoglobin is read at two wavelengths, one at which there is a significant difference between oxy- and deoxyhaemoglobin, the other at the isobestic point of oxy- and deoxyhaemoglobin, the percentage saturation can be obtained. The difference in absorbance between oxygenated and deoxygenated haemoglobin is greatest at 625 nm: 805 nm is the isobestic point of oxyhaemoglobin and deoxyhaemoglobin where the molecular absorption coefficient is the same for both molecules.

The problem of variable tissue absorption was overcome by analysing the pulsatile variations in light absorbance made possible by use of LEDs (light-emitting diodes) as light sources and microprocessor technology to analyse the data.

The pulse oximeter sensor may be placed on the finger, earlobe, nasal septum or toe. It contains two LEDs which emit in the red (about 660 nm) and infrared (about 940 nm) regions of the spectrum, and a photodiode which measures the intensity of the radiation from both LEDs after it has passed through the tissue. In order to be able to identify the absorption at each wavelength, the LEDs are activated sequentially followed by a period when both are off. This sequence is repeated 30 times a second so that the absorption at both wavelengths can be sampled many times during each pulse beat. The result is a steady (DC) signal which depends on the strength of the light source, absorption by the tissues and by the arterial, venous and capillary blood. On this is superimposed a pulsatile signal due to absorbance associated with the greater volume of blood in the light path with each pulsatile wave. The raw signals are then subjected to very complex processing; the resulting ratio of the amplitude of the red/infrared pulsatile signals can then be related to arterial saturation.

Sources of error

These can be summarised as:

* vasoconstriction
* calibration
* delay in response
* interference.

Vasoconstriction

Pulse oximeters become inaccurate when the patient is vasoconstricted from cold, hypovolaemia or in elderly patients with arterial disease. Thus all pulse oximeters should provide an analogue signal of the pulse waveform so that the user can ensure that a satisfactory signal is being obtained.

Calibration

The relationship of red/infrared absorption to saturation is a nonlinear empirical function, so pulse oximeters are usually calibrated by comparing their readings with directly determined arterial saturations in volunteers breathing mixtures containing low concentrations of oxygen. Most of the calibration points are thus in the 80–100% range. Values below 80% are usually extrapolated from the higher readings, and significant errors can occur when reading low saturations.

Delay in response

The delay in pulse oximeter response is due to both instrumental and circulatory delay. In some instruments it can be as long as 10–15 seconds.

Interference

Methylene blue, bilirubin or dark-coloured nail varnish can interfere with the red/infrared signal and lead to error. Large venous pulsations, ambient light, infrared heaters and surgical diathermy can all lead to interference. Fetal haemoglobin has very similar absorption characteristics to adult haemoglobin and will not cause gross errors. If carboxyhaemoglobin (HbCO) is present, the pulse oximeter overestimates the saturation by the percentage of HbCO present. HbCO is normally 3% in urban dwellers but can be as high as 15% in heavy smokers.

Further reading

Barker ST, Tremper KK. The effect of carbon monoxide inhalation on pulse oximeter signal detection. *Anesthesiology* 1987; **67**:599–603.

Cote CJ, Goldstein EA, Fuchsman WM, Hoaglin DC. The effect of nail polish on pulse oximetry. *Anesth Analg* 1988; **67**:683–86.

Hanning CD, Alexander-Williams JM. Pulse oximetry: a practical review. *Br J Anaesth* 1995; **311**:367–70.

Moyle JTB. *Pulse Oximetry*. London: London: BMJ Publishing, 1994.

Severinghaus JW, Naifeh KH. Accuracy of response of six pulse oximeters to profound hypoxia. *Anaesthesiology* 1987; **67**:551–8

Tremper KK, Barker SJ. Pulse oximetry. *Anaesthesiology* 1989; **70**:98–108.

Wilkins CJ, Moores M, Hanning CD. Comparison of pulse oximeters: effects of vasoconstriction and venous engorgement. *Br J Anaesth* 1989; **62**:439–44.

Wukitsch MW, Petterson MT, Tobler D, Polge G. Pulse oximetry: analysis of theory, technology and practice. *J Clin Monitor* 1988; **4**:290–301.

3   Carbon dioxide measurement

> Outline the principles of measurement of carbon dioxide in anaesthetic breathing systems. How may capnography be useful to the anaesthetist?

Principles

An infrared analyser measures carbon dioxide in anaesthetic breathing systems. Infrared radiation in the range $1-15\,\mu m$ is absorbed by all gases with two or more atoms in the molecule provided these atoms are dissimilar. Thus oxygen (O_2) does not absorb infrared radiation but carbon monoxide (CO) does.

Light from an infrared source yielding a wide range of wavelengths is directed down two tubes whose ends are sealed with a substance, which transmits infrared radiation. The gas sample to be analysed is aspirated through the analysis cell whilst the other tube, the reference tube, is flushed with air or other background gas. The gas in the analysis cell absorbs a small proportion of the infrared radiation and the strength of the radiation reaching the detector is therefore less than that impinging on the detector on the reference side.

Clinical uses

Clinical uses of capnography are:
* detection of oesophageal intubation
* disconnection/apnoea alarm
* estimation of P_aCO_2
* monitoring of IPPV and hyperventilation
* detection of reduced end-tidal CO_2 due to physiological upset
* detection of rebreathing
* detection of soda-lime exhaustion
* characteristic capnography displays.

In the conscious patient with healthy lungs, the alveolar plateau of CO_2 approximates closely to arterial PCO_2. When there are ventilation–perfusion inequalities there is an increase in alveolar dead-space and an increase in the arterial to end-tidal PCO_2 difference $(P_{a-A}CO_2)$. When perfusion is reduced the alveolar plateau tends to be horizontal since the non-perfused alveoli empty synchronously with the perfused alveoli. When lung disease is present, however, the well ventilated areas of lung tend to empty early in expiration whilst poorly ventilated areas empty late, so causing an upwardly sloping alveolar plateau.

During anaesthesia in patients with normal lungs, the $P_{a-A}CO_2$ difference averages $0.8\,kPa$. The difference increases during severe hypovolaemia or in patients with severe obstructive airways disease, and it may be as much as

3–4 kPa. The difference is decreased by prolonging inspiration but may increase if alveolar pressure is increased by the use of high positive end-expiratory pressure levels.

Pulmonary embolism causes a flat expiratory plateau lower than the true $P_{a-A}CO_2$ because of dilution of expiratory gases with air from non-perfused alveoli.

Sources of error

There are several sources of error with infrared analysis. There is some overlap in the absorption wavebands of different gases. The fundamental absorption bands for carbon dioxide, nitrous oxide and carbon monoxide are 4.3, 4.5 and 4.7 μm respectively. The absorption spectrum of each gas is quite complex, being centred around the fundamental wavelength, so that overlap is inevitable. As a result, a CO_2 analyser given a sample containing both CO_2 and N_2O will read high, since the N_2O will absorb some infrared energy within the absorption bandwidth for CO_2. This error can be overcome by narrowing the absorption band by special optical filters. A second error arises from 'collision broadening' in which the absorption spectrum of one gas (e.g. CO_2) is actually widened by the physical presence of certain other gases such as nitrogen and N_2O so that absorption is increased. The simplest method of eliminating this error is to calibrate the instrument with gas mixtures that contain the same background gas concentration as that to be analysed.

Modern CO_2 analysers are very stable but should be subjected to a three-point calibration at regular intervals. The infrared radiation is detected by special photocells, and the effect of N_2O is minimised by providing an electrical offset operated by a push-button control. The offset provides a reasonable correction when the N_2O is present at the appropriate concentration (usually 70%) but may not be correct at other concentrations. Recently introduced instruments provide a simultaneous breath-by-breath analysis of CO_2, N_2O and the volatile agents, and correct the problem of interference by using microprocessor technology.

Other exhaled vapours such as ethylalcohol or cyclopropane may cause errors with measured vapour concentrations.

The problem of sampling delay is overcome in some instruments by siting the analysis cell in the airway. The accuracy of most analysers is about +0.1%, in the range 0–10% CO_2.

Further reading

Association of Anaesthetists. *Recommendations for Standards of Monitoring during Anaesthesia and Recovery*. London: AA, 1994.

Brunner JX, Westenskow DR. How the rise time of carbon dioxide analysers influences the accuracy of carbon dioxide measurements. *Br J Anaesth* 1998; **61**:628–38.

McEvoy JDS, Jones NL, Campbell EJM. Mixed venous and arterial P_{CO_2}. *Br Med J* 1974; **4**:687–90.

O'Flaherty D. *Capnography*. London: BMJ Publishing, 1994.

4 Invasive blood pressure measurement

> Describe the physical principles involved in the direct measurement of arterial blood pressure. Discuss the sources of error in this measurement and how they may be reduced.

Clinical applications

Direct measurements of arterial pressure are usually indicated when sudden, large changes of blood volume are expected, such as in major vascular surgery or when rapid and extreme changes in pressure are likely (operation for phaeo-chromocytoma). The shape of the arterial waveform can provide useful information regarding cardiac contractility or aortic valve disease. Direct arterial pressure measurement is further indicated when myocardial function is disturbed by dysrhythmias, myocardial infarction or open-heart surgery, or when non-invasive methods are likely to be inaccurate (obesity or cardiopulmonary bypass).

Principles

Direct measurement of arterial blood pressure requires a catheter placed into the lumen of the artery connected to a pressure transducer by a fluid-filled catheter. The fluid and the mass of the diaphragm represent the oscillating mass, while the compliance of the diaphragm, the tubing and any air bubbles in the system represent the spring.

The problem is that the waveform is complex and not a sine wave as should be the case for simple harmonic motion. All complex waves can be analysed as a mixture of simple sine waves of varying amplitude, frequency and phase. These consist of the fundamental wave (at the pulse frequency) and a series of harmonics. A reasonable approximation to the arterial pressure waveform can often be obtained by accurate reproduction of the fundamental and the first eight to ten harmonics. However, for extremely accurate recording of complex waveforms it is necessary to be able to record a greater range of harmonics. In general, the sharper the waveform the greater the number of harmonics and the higher must be the frequency response.

A recording system must accurately reproduce both the amplitude and phase difference of each harmonic present in the waveform. To achieve this damping, it is necessary to design a system with a high undamped natural frequency or resonant frequency, and then to apply the correct amount. The undamped natural frequency of a mass attached to a spring when in motion is given by the general formula:

$$f_0 = 1/2\pi\sqrt{(S/M)}$$

where f_0 = undamped natural frequency of oscillation, S = stiffness of the spring, and M = mass of the oscillating body. Thus to achieve an undamped natural frequency of oscillation in a system the spring must be stiff and the mass small. In other words the diaphragm of your arterial pressure measurement system must be stiff and the mass of the diaphragm and fluid small.

Thus the undamped resonance frequency of a catheter–transducer measuring system is highest when the velocity of movement of fluid in the catheter is minimised; this is achieved when the diaphragm is stiff and the fluid-containing catheter is short and wide. A short and wide catheter reduces fluid velocity and also offers minimal hindrance to the flow of fluid (Poiseuille's equation), so fluid movement is reduced. It is similarly very important that the catheter has rigid walls, for any elasticity in the catheter will increase the compliance of the whole system and decrease the undamped natural frequency (f_0).

The next important concept to understand is that of critical damping (D). In the undamped state, pressures with a frequency close to the resonant frequency will be exaggerated; whilst in the overdamped state, high-frequency oscillations will be damped out so that the true pressure changes will be underestimated. If the damping of a system is carefully adjusted, a recording can be achieved in which overshoot is minimal and yet the speed of response is only slightly reduced. This point is reached when the overshoot is 7% of the original deflection. The damping is then 64% of critical ($D = 0.64$). This represents the best compromise that can be obtained between speed of response and accuracy of registration of the amplitude of the pressure trace. Optimal damping thus ensures that the maximum use is made of the natural resonant frequency of the system.

Further reading

Allan MWB, Gray WM, Ashburg AJ. Measurement of arterial pressure using catheter–transducer systems: improvement using the Accudynamic. *Br J Anaesth* 1998; **60**:413–18.

Gardner RM. Direct blood pressure management: dynamic response requirements. *Anaesthesiology* 1981; **54**:227–36.

Zorab JSM. Continuous display of the arterial pressure: a simple manometric technique. *Anaesthesia* 1969; **24**:431–7.

5 Temperature measurement

Describe the methods available for measuring body temperature, and detail the physical principles involved.

Principles

Body temperature is normally maintained within a narrow range by *thermoregulation*. Impairment of thermoregulatory mechanisms during anaesthesia contributes to the development of hypothermia, which may have deleterious effects on the patient.

Body temperature can be monitored at a number of different sites:

- rectal
- nasopharyngeal
- oesophageal
- tympanic membrane.

The temperature of the surrounding faeces may affect rectal temperature measurement. There is a small risk of viscous perforation.

Nasopharyngeal temperature reflects brain temperature but may be affected by respiratory gases if the patient is not intubated. Tympanic membrane temperature also reflects brain temperature when closely approximated to the membrane. There is a danger of tympanic membrane perforation and bleeding.

Core temperature is best measured via a pulmonary artery catheter, a urinary catheter incorporating a thermistor or an oesophageal temperature probe.

Skin temperature is dependent on cutaneous blood flow and hence is a poor representation of core temperature. Measuring skin temperature may be useful when measuring the toe-to-core temperature gradient, which is a monitor of adequacy of the circulation in shock or low-output states.

Methods

Temperature is measured using a thermometer, which may measure temperature directly or indirectly:

1. *Direct:*
   liquid expansion
   bimetallic strip
   chemical.
2. *Indirect:*
   resistance wire
   thermistor
   thermocouple.

Liquid expansion thermometers are the simplest and most reliable devices for measuring temperature. The instrument consists of a glass bulb, connected to an evacuated, closed capillary tube. The bulb is filled with a liquid which is generally alcohol or mercury and the temperature is indicated by the position of the meniscus in the capillary tube. This type of thermometer has several disadvantages. It is frail, has a large thermal capacity and so is slow to respond. It is difficult to read and to reset and is unsuitable for insertion into body cavities. It cannot be used for remote reading or recording. Special low-recording thermometers must be used when hypothermia is suspected. It is possible to separate the display from the site of temperature measurement by using liquid or gas expansion thermometers in which the expansion is detected by a pressure-measuring device such as a Bourdon gauge. This type of thermometer is relatively cheap and robust but not very accurate. It is therefore generally employed to measure fairly large temperature changes, such as in humidifiers, water baths and autoclaves.

If strips of two metals with different coefficients of expansion are fastened together throughout their length, the combined bimetallic strip will bend when heated. This principle is used in cheap, but not very accurate thermometers for measuring air temperature. A bimetallic strip is also used in a number of anaesthetic vaporisers to compensate for changes in the temperature of the liquid being vaporised.

Chemical thermometers consist of a strip containing several rows of small cells along its length. Each cell is filled with a unique mixture of chemicals, which melts at a particular temperature, the number of cells being chosen to suit the desired accuracy and temperature range. The chemicals melt within about 30 seconds and, in doing so, release a dye. The temperature is indicated by the number of cells that have changed colour. Reversible chemical thermometers are available.

Resistance-wire thermometers are based on the principle that the resistance of certain metal wires increases as their temperature increases. The metal most commonly used for this purpose is platinum, since it resists corrosion and has a large temperature coefficient of resistance. The resistance change is measured by a battery-operated handpiece, which grips the two terminals at the distal end of the probe.

Thermistors are semiconductors made from the fused oxides of heavy metals such as cobalt, manganese and nickel, and can be made to have positive or negative temperature coefficients. Their resistance varies markedly with temperature but the change is nonlinear. Thermistors have several potential disadvantages. The resistance of individual thermistors in a batch tends to vary. Thermistors tend to 'age' or show a change in resistance with time, and they tend to exhibit hysteresis so that the value of a given temperature recorded during a heating cycle is less than the value recorded at the same temperature during a cooling cycle. An advantage of a thermistor is that, because its temperature coefficient is much greater than that of a resistance-wire element, it can be used to detect very small temperature changes. Furthermore the beads are extremely small and so respond very quickly.

Thermocouple thermometers work on the principle that two dissimilar metals, when joined to create an electrical circuit with the junctions at different temperatures, generate an electrical current from one metal to the other. This phenomenon is known as the Seebeck effect. Common combinations of metals used to make thermocouples are copper–constantan and platinum–rhodium. It is essential to maintain the cold junction at a constant temperature. The advantage of the thermocouple is that all junctions made from the same materials behave identically and are very inexpensive, so that multichannel thermometers can be constructed economically.

6 Perioperative heat loss

> List the factors contributing to heat loss during surgery. How may heat loss be minimised?

Causes of heat loss

During anaesthesia, thermoregulation is impaired and patients are subjected to many thermal stresses. These are due to:

- transfer to theatre
- a cold environment
- exposure of skin
- open body cavities
- cold preparation solutions
- irrigation fluids
- blood
- intravenous fluids
- dry inspired gas
- transfer to the recovery area.

Following induction of anaesthesia, there is an initial drop in temperature of 1°C. Thereafter, body temperature declines at approximately 0–5°C per hour, after which it stabilises at 34–35°C. The initial decrease in temperature occurs as a result of redistribution of heat from the core to peripheral tissues. The subsequent slow decline in temperature is caused by loss of heat to the environment until the loss of heat equals the amount of heat being produced.

General anaesthesia impairs central thermoregulatory control and abolishes behavioural responses. Shivering cannot occur in the presence of neuromuscular blockade. Heat losses to the environment are increased by anaesthetic agents and other drugs which promote vasodilatation. After surgery, body temperature may drop further on transfer to the recovery area and with removal of drapes and the movement of air across the patient.

Minimising heat losses

A number of practical strategies can be employed to avoid patient cooling during surgery:

- warm ambient temperature
- warm intravenous fluids and blood
- warm irrigation fluids
- heated mattress
- covering exposed extremities
- heated air blankets
- humidified inspired gases.

The air temperature in theatre is an important factor. If it is low the patient will lose heat by convection from the skin. The use of heated mattresses and blankets whilst covering the patient up creates a warm 'microclimate'. Warming IV fluids is an important means of preventing heat loss. Humidification of inspired gases avoids heat losses from vaporisation of water.

In recent work an intravenous infusion of a mixture of amino acids suppressed the fall in body temperature due to increased thermogenesis. An increase in cardiorespiratory work is required to support the enhanced energy expenditure needed for this nutrient thermogenesis. This may not be desirable in all patients.

Further reading

Carli F, Macdonald IA. Preoperative inadvertent hypothermia: what do we need to prevent? *Br J Anaesth* 1996; **76**:601–3.

Cooper KE, Kenyon JR. A comparison of temperatures measured in the rectum, oesophagus and on the surface of the aorta during hypothermia in man. *Br J Surg* 1957; **44**:616–19.

Holdcraft A, Hall GM. Heat loss during anaesthesia. *Br J Anaesth* 1978; **50**:157–64.

Imrie MM, Hall GM. Body temperature and anaesthesia. *Br J Anaesth* 1990; **64**:346–54.

Sellden E, Branstrom R, Brundin T. Preoperative infusion of amino acids prevents postoperative hypothermia. *Br J Anaesth* 1996; **76**:227–34.

7 Low-flow anaesthesia

> Discuss the place of low-flow breathing systems in anaesthetic practice. What safeguards would you require when they are used?

A low-flow system refers to a single breathing system in which the fresh gas flow is 3 L/min or less. There are only two low-flow breathing systems: the Waters to-and-fro system and the circle system.

The Waters system

The Waters system consists of an expiratory valve T-piece for fresh gas, soda-lime canister and reservoir bag connected in series. Although widely used in the past, numerous advances have led to its virtual abandonment. The apparatus is bulky and needs to be placed close to the patient's head, causing traction on the endotracheal tube or facemask and so restricting surgical access. There is progressive increase in dead-space as soda-lime nearest to the patient is exhausted. Settlement of soda-lime granules may lead to the formation of a channel between the uppermost part of the soda-lime and the well of the canister through which gas can pass without removal of carbon dioxide. There is furthermore a risk of soda-lime dust inhalation as a consequence of the proximity of the canister to the patient's airway.

The circle system

The circle system is probably the most commonly used breathing system in anaesthesia worldwide. It consists of two unidirectional valves (inspiratory and expiratory), an overflow valve, a reservoir bag, a soda-lime canister and a fresh gas inlet, all connected by tubing.

There are many possible configurations of these components (64 in total). The most efficient system is to position the fresh-gas inlet in the inspired-gas stream proximal to the inspiratory valve. Expired gas is vented via the spill valve upstream of the absorber, conserving soda-lime. The absorber is placed downstream of the overflow valve but before the fresh-gas inlet. Lastly the reservoir bag is positioned upstream of the absorber.

Advantages of the circle system

One advantage of the circle system is the warming of inspired gases by the exothermic reaction of carbon dioxide absorption by soda-lime. This is probably not of great clinical importance except in paediatric anaesthesia. Inspired gases in a low-flow system are nearly 100% saturated with water vapour as a consequence of rebreathing expired gas and water liberated during carbon dioxide absorption, thus avoiding the deleterious effects of dry gas inhalation. The volume of a circle is approximately 5 litres. Thus there is an oxygen reserve in the event of loss of oxygen supply. Low-flow systems undoubtedly reduce operating environmental pollution. Because of much more sparing use of anaesthetic gases and volatile agents, the circle is a very economical breathing system. However, the potential savings in absolute terms are small in comparison with the total cost of providing an anaesthetic service, and negligible in the context of the total cost of healthcare. Against any saving must be offset the cost of purchasing and maintaining additional monitoring equipment needed to use low-flow systems with safety.

Disadvantages of the circle system

There are many disadvantages. A system that is virtually leak-proof is essential with low-flow anaesthesia. Leaks can occur frequently around the seal of the carbon dioxide absorber, so the ability to sustain a pressure in the system must be ensured. At fresh-gas flows of less than 1 L/min, a discrepancy between the vaporiser setting and the inspired concentration of volatile agent by the patient develops. This is because the mass of volatile agent delivered to the system is insufficient to replace anaesthetic taken up by the patient's tissues. At flows exceeding 2 L/min there is negligible difference between inspired concentration and vaporiser setting. With the vaporiser outside the circle the concentration in the circuit cannot increase above that of the vaporiser setting.

One of the biggest disadvantages of the low-flow system is that the anaesthetist is unaware of the inspired gas composition and hence it is advisable to measure volatile agent concentrations. The use of an oxygen monitor is essential when flows of 1 L/min or less are used in the presence of nitrous oxide. The rapid decline in nitrous oxide uptake after the first few minutes of anaesthesia reduces inspired oxygen concentration. Oxygen consumption remains reasonably constant during anaesthesia at approximately 225 mL/min. Nitrous oxide consumption is initially high, but after a period of 20–30 minutes becomes less than that of oxygen. The accumulation of nitrous oxide within the circle at low flows may result in a hypoxic anaesthetic mixture. If fresh-gas flow is 2 L/min or more this problem should not arise.

If a low-flow technique is used from the start of anaesthetic administration, there is a danger of nitrogen accumulation as nitrous oxide is taken up by the patient and nitrogen released. If high fresh-gas flow is used for the first 5 minutes of the anaesthetic, this ensures that nitrogen concentration within the circle is reduced to acceptably low levels of 3–5%.

Summary of advantages and disadvantages of low flow

Advantages:
* Heat conservation.
* Maintenance of humidity.
* O_2 reservoir if failure of supply.
* Decreased pollution.
* Cost saving.

Disadvantages:
* Cost of circle system and soda-lime.
* Complexity of the system.
* Danger of hypoxia.
* Danger of patient awareness.
* Slow changes in depth of anaesthesia.
* Accumulation of anaesthetic metabolites.

Further reading

Barton F, Nunn JF. Totally closed circuit nitrous oxide/oxygen anaesthesia. *Br J Anaesth* 1975; **47**:350–7.

Conway CM. Anaesthetic breathing systems. *Br J Anaesth* 1985; **57**:649–57.

Davey A, Moyle JTB, Ward CS (eds). Breathing systems and their components. In: *Ward's Anaesthetic Equipment*, 3rd edn. London: WB Saunders, 1992, pp. 120–66.

Mapleson WW. The concentration of anaesthetics in closed circuits: I. Theatrical study. *Br J Anaesth* 1960; **32**:298–309.

Spence AA. A guided approach to low-flow anaesthetic systems. In: Zorab J (ed.), *Lectures in Anaesthesiology*, vol. 2. Oxford: Blackwell Scientific, 1986.

Waters RM. Advantages and technique of carbon dioxide filtration with inhalation anaesthesia. *Anaesth Analg* 1926; **3**:160–2.

8 Swan–Ganz catheter

> What can be measured or derived from a successfully placed multi-lumen flow-directed pulmonary artery catheter?

Measured and derived values

1. *Measured values:*
   Pulmonary artery pressures (systolic and diastolic).
   Pulmonary artery wedge pressure.
   Cardiac output.
   Mixed venous oxygen saturation.
   Right heart pressure (CVP).

2. *Derived values:*
   Stroke volume.
   Systemic vascular resistance.
   Pulmonary vascular resistance.
   Left cardiac work.
   Right cardiac work.

Using the Swan–Ganz catheter

A multi-lumen flow-directed pulmonary artery catheter (PA catheter) – or Swan–Ganz catheter – may provide valuable information to assess left ventricular function, to measure pressures in the left side of the heart, to optimise left ventricular filling pressure, and to allow thermal dilution cardiac output measurements to be made.

The catheter is passed through a sheath inserted into a central vein and threaded into a position near the right atrium. The balloon is then inflated with the recommended volume of air and the catheter advanced. The balloon is carried in the direction of the blood flow and so passes through the right atrium and right ventricle into the pulmonary artery, the position being detected by observation of the pressure trace.

Measurement of pulmonary artery pressures identifies pulmonary hypertension. In the absence of increased pulmonary resistance the pulmonary artery end-diastolic pressure (PAEDP) is about 1–3 mmHg higher than the pulmonary artery wedge pressure (PAWP). Poor correlation between the central venous pressure (CVP) and PAWP has been demonstrated in critically ill patients. In this situation the PAWP may be preferable for assessment of fluid management.

PAWP gives an indirect measurement of the left atrial pressure (LAP) which equates to the left ventricular end-diastolic pressure (LVEDP). The major source of error with the wedge measurement is the position of the catheter. If the tip is wedged in the upper zones of the lung there may be no fluid connection between the catheter and left atrium, since alveolar pressure may exceed capillary pressure. The area of lung subjected to these conditions may be increased if positive end-expiratory pressure (PEEP) is applied so that the pressure recorded may be alveolar rather than left atrial. It is therefore important to check that the catheter tip lies in the lower lung zones, by observing its position on a chest x-ray, and to take all readings at the end of expiration whether ventilation is spontaneous or controlled. The normal PAWP is 8–12 mmHg. The mean PAWP correlates well with LVEDP over a wide range of filling pressures in patients who have normal left ventricular and mitral valve function but may be greater than LVEDP when there is mitral stenosis, left atrial myxoma or during application of PEEP. In left ventricular failure the elevated LVEDP may exceed the mean left atrial and mean PAWP.

Thermal-dilution cardiac output measurements can be made repeatedly, and automated analysis of the curve recorded from a thermistor in the pulmonary artery can yield a value for cardiac output within seconds of injection. A temperature versus time thermal-dilution curve is constructed, the area under the curve is computed by integration, and this is inversely proportional to cardiac output.

The accuracy of the thermal technique is critically dependent on the time of injection during the respiratory cycle, variations of up to 50% of the value being obtained between injections made during the inspiratory or expiratory phases of mechanical ventilation. To minimise this error, injections are made at end-expiration.

Mixed venous saturation measurements are most useful when there are acute changes in the circulation. Continuous monitoring detects acute falls in saturation due to transient increases in oxygen consumption. A fall in mixed venous oxygen saturation, in the absence of increased tissue oxygen consumption, is an indication of decreased cardiac output. Values greater than 60% generally imply satisfactory cardiac output while values below 40% suggest significant inadequacy of oxygen delivery. The mixed venous saturation value is affected not only by the relationship of oxygen consumption to cardiac output, but also by all the factors which affect the supply of oxygen to the tissues – such as inspired oxygen fraction, ventilation, haemoglobin concentration, oxygen dissociation curve and abnormal haemoglobin. Furthermore, in situations where marked vasoconstriction exists, the mixed venous saturation may be normal despite a severe fall in cardiac output because much of the tissue mass is not being perfused.

Stroke volume measures the amount of blood ejected by the ventricle with each cardiac contraction. It is calculated by dividing the cardiac output by the heart rate. Stroke volume is 60–70 mL (normal range for stroke index is 41–51 mL/m^2). The stroke volume depends on factors affecting the preload, afterload and myocardial contractility.

Systemic vascular resistance measures the load applied to the left ventricular muscle during ventricular ejection. Vascular resistance to blood flow is calculated by analogy to Ohm's law, which states for an electrical circuit:

Resistance equals *voltage difference* divided by *current flow*.

Similarly for vascular resistance:

Resistance equals *mean pressure differential across vascular bed* divided by *blood flow*.

The pressure difference between the proximal and distal ends of the cardiovascular system (arteriovenous) is divided by the cardiac output. This value is multiplied by the conversion factor of 79.96 which changes resistance units of mmHg/L/min to dyne.s/cm^5.

Pulmonary vascular resistance is an index of the resistance offered by the pulmonary capillaries to the systolic effort of the right ventricle. As with SVR, PVR is calculated by analogy to Ohm's law by deriving the pressure differential between the mean pulmonary arterial pressure and pulmonary artery wedge pressure and dividing that value by the cardiac output. So:

$$\text{PVR [dyne.s/cm}^5] = 79.96 \times (\text{PAP}_m - \text{PAWP})/\text{CO}$$

Under normal circumstances, the pulmonary vascular resistance is one-sixth that of the systemic vascular bed. Pulmonary vascular disease is associated with increased PVR, which may exceed SVR. In normal lungs, pulmonary artery pressures do not increase until approximately two-thirds of the lung vessels are obstructed.

Work is measured as the product of a force and the distance moved by the point of application of that force. Thus cardiac work is the product of pressure generated and volume of blood pumped:

Work is *pressure generated* multiplied by *volume of blood pumped*.

LCW (left cardiac work) measures the amount of work the left ventricle does each minute when ejecting blood. Arterial work is not included because of the relatively small pressures involved. Left cardiac work is the product of the mean arterial blood pressure and the cardiac output. The conversion factor of 0.0136 converts mmHg to kg.m.

Left ventricle stroke work is LCW divided by heart rate or the product of stroke volume and mean arterial blood pressure:

$$\text{LCW [kg.m]} = \text{CO} \times \text{ABP}_m \times 0.0136.$$

Similarly, *right cardiac work* (RCW) measures the work that the right ventricle does each minute when ejecting blood. It is calculated as the product of the mean pulmonary artery pressure and the cardiac output:

$$RCW \text{ [kg.m]} = CO \times PAP_m \times 0.0136.$$

Right ventricular stroke work (RVSW) measures the amount of work the right ventricle does per beat when ejecting blood, similar to the left ventricular stroke work measurement. It is calculated as the product of the mean pulmonary artery pressure and the stroke volume or RCW divided by heart rate.

Further reading

Bedford RF. Invasive blood pressure monitoring. In: Blitt CD (ed.), *Monitoring in Anaesthesia and Critical Care Medicine*, 2nd edn. London: Churchill Livingstone, 1990, 93–134.

Buchbinder N, Ganz W. Hemodynamic monitoring: invasive techniques. *Anaesthesiology* 1976; **45**:146–55.

Hansen PM *et al*. Poor correlation between pulmonary arterial wedge pressure and left ventricular end-diastolic volume after coronary bypass graft surgery. *Anaesthesiology* 1986; **64**:764–70.

Kaplin JA, Wells PM. Early diagnosis of myocardial ischaemia using the pulmonary arterial catheter. *Anaesth Analg* 1981; **60**:789–93.

Nadeau S, Noble WH. Misinterpretation of pressure measurements from the pulmonary artery catheter. *Can Anaesth Soc J* 1986; **33**:352–63.

Pierce T, Woodcock T. How to insert a pulmonary arterial flotation catheter. *Br J Hosp Med* 1989; **42**:484–7.

Multiple-choice questions: Physics

1. During a long operation, reliable monitors of core temperatures include:
   a) a temperature probe at the tympanic membrane
   b) a temperature probe in the rectum
   c) a quadriceps muscle temperature
   d) a temperature probe in the nasopharynx
   e) a temperature probe in the oesophagus at the level of the cricoid.

2. Blood pressure measured by an automatic non-invasive method:
   a) may over-read at high pressure
   b) may over-read at low pressure
   c) is affected by arrhythmias
   d) may cause ulnar nerve damage
   e) cuff width does not affect the measurement.

3. A saline manometer inserted via the antecubital fossa for CVP measurement should:
   a) not be longer than 20 cm
   b) have an ideal diameter of 0.25 mm
   c) be measured from the angle of Louis whatever the position of the patient
   d) is best inserted by the cephalic vein
   e) have less infection risk than a catheter placed in the internal jugular vein.

4. Methods of measuring halothane in an anaesthetic breathing system include:
   a) gas chromatography
   b) mass spectrometry
   c) ultraviolet spectrometry
   d) infrared spectrometry
   e) refractometry.

5. Concerning the respiratory function tests:
   a) the pneumotachograph is suitable for measuring peak flow
   b) peak flow can be determined from a vitalograph
   c) FEV_1/FVC decreases with obstructive disease
   d) airway resistance can be measured by plethysmography
   e) dynamic compliance decreases as respiratory rate increases.

6. The saturated vapour pressure (SVP) of water:
   a) is zero at 273 K
   b) is the same as blood at 37°C
   c) is equal to atmospheric pressure at 100°C
   d) is dependent on altitude
   e) is altered by solutes in the water.

7. Regarding the flow directed multi-lumen pulmonary artery (PA) catheter:
   a) the thermistor is situated 20 cm from the tip
   b) pulmonary capillary wedge is a small bronchopulmonary segment
   c) cardiac estimations can be performed by pressure measurement
   d) an open central lumen when the balloon is inflated protects against distal infarction
   e) is more accurate when inserted via the internal jugular vein than via the subclavian vein.

8. In the Severinghaus electrode:
   a) the electrolyte solution is sodium bicarbonate surrounding a pH-sensitive electrode
   b) contains carbon dioxide-sensitive gas
   c) is affected by temperature
   d) is more accurate for blood than gas sample analysis
   e) is affected by nitrous oxide.

9. Regarding the measurement of an anaesthetic agent:
   a) infrared measurement is agent-specific
   b) mass spectrometry is not agent-specific
   c) nitrous oxide interferes with paramagnetic analysers
   d) acoustics can be used for measurement
   e) infrared analysers pick up isopropyl alcohol.

10. Regarding pulmonary artery catheters in a normal person:
    a) the wedge pressure is about 12 mmHg
    b) the pulmonary artery pressure is about 20/5 mmHg
    c) the CVP is about 5 cmH$_2$O
    d) the right ventricular pressure is about 30/0 mmHg
    e) the internal jugular to wedged distance is about 70 cm.

11. To measure right to left shunt the following are needed:
    a) end capillary P_{O_2}
    b) mixed venous P_{O_2}
    c) arterial P_{O_2}
    d) cardiac output
    e) oxygen saturation.

12. The following can be measured with a dry spirometer:
    a) expiratory reserve volume (ERV)
    b) functional residual capacity (FRC)
    c) closing volume
    d) total lung capacity (TLC)
    e) tidal volume (TV).

13. Critical temperature of a gas is that:
    a) at which the pressure is the critical pressure
    b) at which freezing takes place
    c) at which attraction between gas molecules is negligible
    d) above which the gas cannot be ignited
    e) at which Boyle's law is perfectly obeyed.

14. When using a vaporiser outside a circle system (VOC):
    a) the vaporiser is usually temperature-compensated
    b) the temperature of the agent in the vaporiser rises with an increase in fresh gas flow
    c) the vapour pressure of the agent is inversely proportional to the temperature
    d) the inspired concentration of the volatile agent is a function of alveolar ventilation
    e) the alveolar concentration is a function of pulmonary perfusion.

15. An electrical potential difference between two points:
    a) is a measure of the electric field intensity in that region
    b) describes the electrical energy difference between those points
    c) is measured in volts
    d) is measured in volts/m
    e) depends on the square of the local current flow.

16. The resistance of the cylindrical conductor
    a) increases with increasing length
    b) increases with decreasing cross-sectional area
    c) depends upon the dielectric constant of the conductor material
    d) decreases at higher temperature
    e) is reciprocally related to the conductance.

17. Which of the following has a critical temperature which is negative on the celsius scale?
    a) nitrous oxide
    b) entonox
    c) carbon dioxide
    d) oxygen
    e) cyclopropane.

18. A volatile liquid is allowed to equilibrate with a mixture of gases. The resulting partial pressure of the vapour will depend on:
    a) atmospheric pressure
    b) ambient temperature
    c) the surface area of the liquid
    d) the volume of liquid
    e) the composition of the mixture of gases.

19. Infrared gas analysis can be used to measure:
    a) nitrous oxide
    b) oxygen
    c) halothane
    d) carbon dioxide
    e) trichloroethylene.
20. Turbulent flow of gas through a tube is related to:
    a) length of the tube
    b) pressure difference across the tube
    c) viscosity of the gas
    d) density of the gas
    e) radius of the tube.
21. The pressure gauge on a nitrous oxide cylinder reads 5000 kPa. It may be:
    a) quarter full
    b) half full
    c) three-quarters full
    d) full
    e) supplying 5 L/min.
22. The volume displacement of an electromanometer:
    a) indicates the amount of liquid needed to fill it
    b) depends on the volume of the chamber
    c) depend on the stiffness of the diaphragm
    d) depends on the frequency of the response
    e) is not affected by the radius of the measurement catheter.
23. Body temperature can be measured by:
    a) galvanic skin resistance
    b) small metal wire resistance
    c) a hot-wire anemometer
    d) a thermistor
    e) a thermocouple.
24. Radiation is the emission of:
    a) beta particles
    b) alpha particles
    c) neutrons
    d) gamma rays
    e) any waveform.

25. For the Fick method of measurement of cardiac output, the following are needed:
    a) respiratory quotient
    b) oxygen uptake
    c) oxygen content arterial blood
    d) oxygen content mixed venous blood
    e) P_aCO_2.
26. The following statements regarding monitoring are correct:
    a) an end-tidal carbon dioxide concentration of 4 kPa excludes rebreathing during spontaneous ventilation
    b) a pulmonary capillary wedge pressure (PCWP) >13 mmHg indicates over-transfusion
    c) the EEG indicates depth of anaesthesia
    d) a small blood pressure cuff over-reads
    e) increased beat to beat variability occurs in hypervolaemia.
27. Pulse oximetry:
    a) the alarm should be set at an oxygen saturation of 85%
    b) is affected by bilirubin
    c) is inaccurate with an oxygen saturation less than 70%
    d) is affected by incident light
    e) is affected by carboxyhaemoglobin.

Answers to multiple-choice questions

1.	a) True;	b) False;	c) False;	d) True;	e) False
2.	a) False;	b) True;	c) True;	d) True;	e) False
3.	a) False;	b) False;	c) False;	d) False;	e) False
4.	a) False;	b) True;	c) True;	d) True;	e) True
5.	a) True;	b) True;	c) True;	d) True;	e) True
6.	a) True;	b) False;	c) True;	d) False;	e) True
7.	a) False;	b) False;	c) False;	d) False;	e) False
8.	a) True;	b) False;	c) True;	d) False;	e) False
9.	a) True;	b) False;	c) False;	d) True;	e) True
10.	a) True;	b) False;	c) True;	d) False;	e) False
11.	a) True;	b) True;	c) True;	d) False;	e) True
12.	a) True;	b) False;	c) False;	d) False;	e) True
13.	a) False;	b) False;	c) False;	d) False;	e) False
14.	a) True;	b) False;	c) False;	d) True;	e) True
15.	a) False;	b) True;	c) True;	d) False;	e) False
16.	a) True;	b) True;	c) False;	d) False;	e) True
17.	a) False;	b) True;	c) False;	d) True;	e) False
18.	a) False;	b) True;	c) False;	d) False;	e) False
19.	a) True;	b) False;	c) True;	d) True;	e) True
20.	a) True;	b) True;	c) True;	d) True;	e) True
21.	a) True;	b) True;	c) True;	d) True;	e) True
22.	a) False;	b) True;	c) True;	d) False;	e) False
23.	a) True;	b) True;	c) False;	d) False;	e) True
24.	a) True;	b) True;	c) True;	d) True;	e) False
25.	a) False;	b) True;	c) True;	d) True;	e) False
26.	a) False;	b) False;	c) True;	d) True;	e) False
27.	a) False;	b) True;	c) True;	d) True;	e) True

SPECIAL CLINICAL PROBLEMS

1 Non-cardiac surgery after heart transplant

A 35-year-old man had a heart transplant four years ago. He is now troubled by pain from avascular necrosis of the head of femur, and requires surgery. He is on cyclosporin, azathioprine and prednisolone. What are the implications of his immunosuppressive treatment for perioperative anaesthesia care?

Complications of cardiac transplantation

One- and 10-year survival rates for cardiac transplantation are 90% and 50% respectively. Fifty per cent of recipients are aged 50 years or over at the time of transplantation.

The main complications of cardiac transplantation encountered in anaesthesia for non-cardiac surgery are:
- donor coronary artery disease
- rejection
- immunosuppression.

Donor coronary artery disease

This is the major long-term medical complication and is the most common cause of death after the first year. Coronary artery disease in this group of patients is immunologically mediated; it is microvascular in origin, only involving proximal vessels when far advanced. Patients do not normally present with angina as the heart is denervated. Instead they present with left ventricular dysfunction or arrhythmia. It is therefore essential that coronary perfusion pressures be maintained during anaesthesia.

Rejection

Acute rejection is uncommon after the first year of transplantation when patients are on stable immunosuppressive treatment. Unexplained weight gain, pyrexia, deterioration in graft function or fluid retention can be signs and symptoms of graft rejection.

Immunosuppression

Long-term treatment based on cyclosporin, azathioprine and prednisolone forms the basis of immunosuppression. Complications include infection, musculoskeletal problems, chronic renal impairment and increased incidence of malignancy. Immunosuppressive medications have pre-, intra- and postoperative implications related to their actions and side-effect profiles.

Preoperative implications

In addition to a full history and examination, side-effects of the immunosuppressant drugs should be looked for:

- *Cyclosporin:*
  - immunosuppression
  - skin cancers, lymphomas
  - hypertension (occurs in 80% of patients, and requires aggressive therapy)
  - nephrotoxicity (common with cyclosporin, related to interstitial fibrosis).
- *Azathioprine:*
  - bone marrow suppression may require pre-op blood transfusion
  - peripheral neuropathies.
- *Steroids:*
  - immunosuppression
  - osteoporosis
  - fat-deposition changes
  - diabetes mellitus/glucose intolerance
  - skin changes
  - adrenal suppression.

Investigations should include:
- FBC
- urea, creatinine and electrolytes
- ECG
- chest x-ray
- cyclosporin levels.

Intraoperative implications

There will be susceptibility to infections, so use alcohol and betadine for access/lines. Take care with intravenous fluids, perioperative prophylactic antibiotics, and circuit filters on the breathing circuit.

The patient will require supplemental intravenous steroids to cover the maintenance 'stress response', to physiologically match the adrenal response to stress (e.g. IV hydrocortisone 50 mg q.i.d.). This should continue until oral intake (maintenance) and a 48-hours tapered dose.

Intravenous cyclosporin will occasionally be required while the patient is 'nil by mouth'. There is a risk of an anaphylactoid reaction to the preparation.

Care should be taken with positioning of the patient, owing to osteoporosis and the neuropathy risk.

Monitor renal function carefully (urine output). Finally, be aware of the sympathectomised heart.

Postoperative implications

These include:

- meticulous fluid management
- return to preoperative doses of medication as soon as possible
- good pain management
- management in a high-dependency unit.

Further reading

Sharpe MD. Anaesthesia and the transplanted patient. *Can J Anaesth* 1996; **43**:R89–93.

Shaw IH, Kirk AJB, Conacher ID. Anaesthesia for patients with transplanted hearts and lungs undergoing non-cardiac surgery. *Br J Anaesth* 1991; **67**:772–8.

2 Septoplasty

An obese 40-year-old man with a history of snoring presents for septoplasty and cautery of turbinates. Describe the anaesthetic management of this patient.

Full history

Snoring at night (reported by bed partner)
1. Is it associated with cessation of breathing/cyanosis?
2. Is there awakening through the night?
3. Is there daytime sleepiness even when talking to others?
4. Morning headache may signify overnight hypoxia or hypercarbia.
5. Has a sleep study been done in the past? If so, what was the score (see below)?
    On nocturnal continuous positive airway pressure (CPAP) at home?
    Previous treatment for obstructive sleep apnoea (OSA) – uvuloplasty?

Apnoea score
*   Apnoea >10 seconds = true apnoea.
*   Apnoea <10 seconds = hypopnoea.
Score apnoea or hypopnoea per hour:
1. If >10 = obstructive sleep anoea.
2. If >20–30 = severe.

Associated conditions

Cor pulmonale
OSA may lead to, or contribute to, cor pulmonale. Ask about:
*   fatigue or exertion
*   peripheral oedema
*   orthopnoea.

Hypertension
Ask about previous checks, treatment and any associated conditions:
*   angina
*   left ventricular failure (LVF)
*   renal condition.

Other
Enquire about:
*   neurobehavioural problems (as mentioned above)
*   recurrent upper respiratory tract infections

- alcohol use
- obesity
- hay fever/vasomotor rhinitis
- craniofacial abnormalities
- macroglossia.

Examination

- Weight.
- Head and neck:
    - airway abnormalities
    - obesity
    - Mallampati classification
    - mandibular size
    - neck mobility
    - oropharynx
    - enlarged tongue.
- Blood pressure.
- Signs of right ventricular failure:
    - right ventricular heave
    - raised jugular venous pressure
    - tricuspid regurgitation murmur
    - peripheral oedema
    - respiratory crepitations.
- Signs of left ventricular failure:
    - tachycardia
    - displaced apex beat
    - murmur of aortic stenosis or regurgitation.

Preoperative investigations

- FBC.
- Chest x-ray.
- ECG.
- Urea and electrolytes.
- Liver function tests.
- Arterial blood gases on air.

Apnoea/hypopnoea index (AHI)

This index is the number of apnoea and/or hypopnoea occurrences per hour of sleep. If AHI ≥70 and the lowest saturation is 80%, *this is highly predictive of perioperative airway complications.*

Anaesthetic technique

1. No premedicant is given. Sleep apnoea patients are very sensitive to even a small dose of benzodiazepine or opioid.
2. Give antacid, H_2 antagonists and metoclopramide.
3. Give an anticholinergic if awake intubation is planned.
4. Monitoring to include:
    ECG (including lead V5)
    arterial line in the morbidly obese in all but the shortest cases
    pulse oximetry
    capnography
    IV access.

Airway management

- Equipment must be able to cope with the patient's weight.
- A powerful ventilator may be needed.
- Endotracheal intubation may be necessary because other means of maintaining the airway are very difficult. There is a high incidence of difficult intubation in morbidly obese patients.
- Use intermittent positive-pressure ventilation (IPPV) because of the risk of hypoventilation and aspiration.
- Consider awake fibreoptic intubation.
- Consider general anaesthesia with rapid-sequence induction. Large induction doses are needed.
- Neuromuscular block must be fully reversed and the patient awake with protective upper airway reflexes intact before extubation.

Postoperative management

Consider elective admission to the intensive-care or high-dependency unit because of the high risk of cardiorespiratory complications in morbidly obese patients.

There is a high incidence of deep vein thrombosis (DVT), so prophylactic measures are recommended.

Further reading

Chambers WA. ENT anaesthesia. In: Nimmo WS, Rowbotham DJ, Smith G (eds), *Anaesthesia*, 2nd edn. London: Blackwell Scientific, 1994, pp. 806–22.

Shenkman Z, Shir Y, Brodsky JB. Perioperative management of the obese patient. *Br J Anaesth* 1993; **70**:349–59.

3 Monitoring in magnetic resonance imaging (MRI)

> What are the problems of monitoring anaesthetised patients in the magnetic resonance imaging unit?

Magnetic resonance imaging (MRI) requires the generation of a very strong magnetic field which aligns protons in a cell along the axis of the electromagnetic field. It is the presence of this strong magnetic field within the MRI scanning room that causes problems with monitoring. Some are listed below.

1. Patients are often children.
2. Patients are anaesthetised in remote areas often a long way from the theatre complex.
3. The patient is enclosed in a long narrow tube where access is difficult.
4. Patients are often anaesthetised in a separate room next to the scanner and are then transferred into the scanner. Monitoring used in the scanner must be non-ferrous. The magnetic field would induce current within electrical cabling with consequent heating, leading to thermal injury in the patient.
5. All ferrous objects within the MRI room will be attracted to the magnet. If close to the field these objects become projectiles.
6. Anaesthetic machines containing ferrous metals must remain outside the magnetic field. Metallic objects within the magnetic field may interfere with the image generated. Non-magnetic anaesthetic machines and gas cylinders are available but very expensive.
7. Long sampling and monitoring leads and anaesthetic tubing are required to reach the patient. The maximum distance the patient moves into the tunnel must be allowed for prior to scanning. There is consequent delayed gas sampling time due to long tubing.
8. Infusion pumps may malfunction or fail if placed within the magnetic field.
9. Special non-ferrous ECG electrodes and pulse oximeter probes and cables are required that are MRI-compatible.
10. If the patient contains metal (cardiac pacemaker, plated bones etc.) this will interefere with the image. Pacemakers will malfunction within magnetic fields.

4   Subtotal thyroidectomy

List and discuss the perioperative complications of subtotal thyroidectomy.

Thyroid disease presents the most common endocrine disorder after diabetes mellitus. Anaesthetists will encounter patients with thyroid disorders presenting for thyroid surgery. The prevalence of hyperthyroidism is 1.9% in females compared to 0.16–0.23% in males. The prevalence of overt hypothyroidism is 1.4% in females and less than 0.1% in males.

Complications

- *Preoperative assessment:*
  - ? hyperthyroidism
  - ? hypothyroidism
  - ? goitre.
- *Intraoperative management:*
  - hyperthyroidism
  - hypothyroidism
  - airway.
- *Postoperative complications:*
  - bleeding
  - vocal cord paralysis
  - hypocalcaemia
  - airway obstruction
  - metabolic abnormality
  - thyroid metabolic emergency.

Hyperthyroidism

The three most common causes of hyperthyroidism are Graves' disease, toxic multinodular goitre and toxic adenoma. Other causes include:
- subacute, postpartum and painless thyroiditis
- drug-induced (iodine, thyroxine and amiodarone)
- thyrotropin (TSH) secreting tumour
- stroma ovarii
- metastatic follicular carcinoma.

Thyrotoxicosis in the context of Graves' disease is most common in women aged 30–50 years. The patient usually presents with symptoms of several months' duration. The most common symptoms are:
- loss of weight despite a normal or increased appetite
- palpitations
- dyspnoea on exertion

- emotional lability
- intolerance to heat
- increased sweating
- fatigue
- menstrual abnormalities.

The patient appears thin, nervous and hyperactive with warm, moist skin. Other signs include a goitre with or without bruit, exopthalmos, lid retraction, hyperkinesis, fine finger tremor, tachycardia and arrhythmias. Symptoms of opthalmopathy are present in 50% of patients and may range from a mild sensation of grittiness to severe periorbital swelling and protrusion of the eyes, diplopia and visual loss from compression of the optic nerve or scarring from the cornea.

The apathetic form of hyperthyroidism is most commonly seen in the elderly (but can occur at any age) and their illness often features absence of hyperkinesis, confusion, depression, greater weight loss, cardiovascular dysfunction with atrial fibrillation and severe proximal myopathy.

Hyperthyroid patients should be rendered euthyroid preoperatively using antithyroid drugs. Alternatively, long-acting propranolol may be used for the preparation of hyperthyroid patients, alone or together with potassium iodide. Their advantage is a much shorter preparation time preoperatively, and they may also be used in patients who are allergic to carbimazole and propylthiouracil. Propanalol acts by blocking the peripheral adrenergic effects of the thyronines and also by inhibiting the deiodination of T4 and thus reducing plasma T3 levels. The half-life of thyroxine is 7 days, so β blockade must be maintained immediately postoperatively and continued for at least 7 days to prevent thyroid crisis. When on beta-blockers the patient should be fully β-blocked and the resting pulse rate should be below 90 bpm before surgery. Potassium iodide is added to the beta-blocker for 7–10 days preoperatively to reduce the circulating thyroid hormone level to within normal range. The iodides inhibit the release of T4 by the thyroid gland but have only a temporary effect. Potassium iodide may be used as the sole agent in emergency situations if beta-blockers are contraindicated. Thyrotoxicosis may be complicated by atrial fibrillation in 10–30% of patients, and 10–40% of patients with thyrotoxic atrial fibrillation have had embolic events, the majority of which are cerebral. The prevalence of thyrotoxic atrial fibrillation increases with age and is more common in men.

Hypothyroidism

In 90% of cases primary hypothyroidism is caused by:

- spontaneous atrophic thyroiditis
- Hashimoto's thyroiditis
- treatment of hyperthyroidism
- lithium carbonate
- excess intake of iodides

- iodine deficiency
- failure of thyroid hormone synthesis due to secondary thyroid failure due to hypothalamic–pituitary disease.

The onset of hypothyroidism is usually insidious with weight gain, a general slowing down and cold intolerance being the most common complaints. Alopecia, hoarseness of voice, depression, bradycardia and hyperlipidaemia are other features. The patient may be overweight with dry skin, coarse hair with loss of the outer one third of the eyebrows, puffy face, yellowish pallor and delayed reflexes. A goitre may be present in Hashimoto's thyroiditis. Younger patients may be totally asymptomatic, despite severe hypothyroidism.

After starting thyroxine sodium treatment (25–50 μg daily), symptomatic improvement is seen in 2–3 weeks, but it takes 6 weeks of full-dose treatment for serum TSH levels to return to normal. Patients with ischaemic heart disease may develop angina when treatment is commenced and thus concomitant anti-anginal treatment is given as necessary. It may be necessary for the patient to have coronary angioplasty or cardiac bypass graft surgery before full replacement can be achieved.

Hypothyroid patients are at increased risk during anaesthesia and surgery and should be rendered euthyroid before any elective procedure is performed. Careful preoperative assessment and investigation will help to detect previously undiagnosed cases. Oral thyroxine takes up to 10 days to exert its maximum effect, whereas oral tri-iodothyronine (T3) acts within 6 hours and exerts its maximal effect in 48–72 hours.

Hypothyroid patients have a higher prevalence of preoperative risk factors, such as anaemia and hypertension. Presence of hoarseness, slurred speech and macroglossia indicates infiltration of the tissues by mucopolysaccharides. Choking and stridor indicate upper-airway obstruction and possible difficult intubation. Delayed gastric emptying, decreased peristalsis, silent gastrointestinal bleeding and ascites are associated with severe hypothyroidism. Chronic peripheral vasoconstriction in hypothyroidism results in significant reduction in blood volume.

Preoperative investigations include:

- ECG
- chest x-ray
- lung function tests
- CT scan
- vocal cords.

The ECG changes include sinus bradycardia, alterations of the ST segment, flattened or inverted T waves, prolongation of the PR interval and low voltage of the QRS complexes, P and T waves. Pericardial effusion is probably responsible in part for the changes. (In hyperthyroidism, sinus tachycardia or supraventricular arryrhmias, especially atrial fibrillation, is seen.)

Chest x-ray reveals the presence of cardiomegaly, cardiac failure, and pleural and pericardial effusions. In patients with suspected retrosternal extension, chest x-rays with thoracic inlet views are performed. In the presence of substernal goitres, PA and lateral views of the chest may show tracheal deviation, soft tissue mass or calcification.

Lung function tests should be requested in patients who have a goitre producing pressure symptoms. Flow volume loop is the best means of identifying upper-airway obstruction; measurement of the peak expiratory flow on its own is not sensitive enough for routine clinical purposes. Flow volume loops help to identify the site of obstruction (intrathoracic and extrathoracic) and help to differentiate airway distress related to thyroid pressure from that of chronic obstructive airway disease or asthma.

A computerised tomography (CT) scan is useful if upper-airway obstruction is suspected, and scans are more reliable than chest x-rays in evaluating tracheal diameters at the zone of tracheal narrowing. However, it may be hazardous to carry out this investigation in patients with acute respiratory compromise. Magnetic resonance imaging (MRI) is helpful if the lesion extends below the clavicle, and ultrasonography (US) can be used to visualise the extent of the goitre if the lesion is confined to the neck.

Preoperative vocal cord examination is carried out routinely in patients having thyroid surgery for medicolegal purposes. Indirect laryngoscopy determines the position of the larynx and so helps to assure a smooth intubation.

Intraoperative management

Tracheal intubation using an armoured endotracheal tube is the usual practice in thyroid surgery. There have been reports where laryngeal mask airways (LMAs) have been used successfully to maintain the airway in thyroid surgery. The advantage of using this technique is that a fibreoptic bronchoscope can be passed through the laryngeal mask airway to visualise the cord movement when the recurrent laryngeal nerve is electrically stimulated. The disadvantages are displacement of the laryngeal mask airway during surgery, laryngeal spasm and insufficient seal between the LMA and the larynx.

Care should be taken to protect the eyes, especially in the presence of exopthalmos, prior to the placement of head towels. The anaesthetic breathing system should be securely attached to the tracheal tube connector, as this will be inaccessible during the operation. A reverse Trendelenberg position aids venous drainage and reduces blood loss in the field. This heightens the risk of air embolus.

Postoperative complications

Postoperative haemorrhage is a serious but uncommon complication of thyroidectomy. Haematoma developing deep to the pretracheal muscles may be fatal. Close observation and early intervention are required. The risk can be minimised by good haemostasis prior to wound closure, avoidance of coughing, elevation of the head of the bed by 30 degrees, and compressive neck dressing.

Damage to the recurrent laryngeal nerve may be unilateral or bilateral, temporary or permanent. In transient palsy, recovery of nerve functions occurs within 3 months. If the nerve has not been identified at surgery then paralysis will be permanent in up to one-third of the injured nerves. Examination of the vocal cords at the time of extubation using direct laryngoscopy is unreliable; indirect laryngoscopy on the third or fourth postoperative day will confirm if both vocal cords are functioning. Alternative methods to visualise the cords have been suggested: the tracheal tube is withdrawn over a fibreoptic bronchoscope when normal ventilatory pattern has been established; by using a fibreoptic nasolaryngoscope; and by passing a fibreoptic bronchoscope through a laryngeal mask airway and stimulating the nerve electrically. Unilateral recurrent laryngeal nerve injury results in hoarseness of voice, while bilateral injury results in aphonia requiring urgent intubation.

Hypocalcaemia may occur as a result of damage or impairment of the blood supply to the parathyroid glands and it may be transient or permanent. Daily serum calcium should be determined and hypocalcaemia treated if the patient is symptomatic or if the serum calcium level drops below 1.6 mmol/L.

An expanding haematoma, tracheomalacia, bilateral recurrent laryngeal nerve palsy and laryngeal mucosal oedema due to venous and lymphatic obstruction resulting from operative manipulation of the trachea may cause airway obstruction.

Thyroid storm is a life-threatening exacerbation of the hyperthyroid state seen usually in association with Graves' disease or toxic multinodular goitre, in which there is multisystem dysfunction. It is associated with a high mortality rate. In most cases of thyroid storm, a precipitating event can be identified; they include:

- infection
- thyroidal and non-thyroidal surgery
- radio-iodine therapy
- diabetic ketoacidosis
- pulmonary embolism
- parturition
- cerebrovascular event
- pre-eclamptic toxaemia
- trauma.

The clinical features are those of thyrotoxicosis, but are severe and exaggerated and include hyperpyrexia, tachyarrhythmias, high-output cardiac failure, cardiovascular collapse, severe agitation, delirium, stupor and coma. Gastrointestinal symptoms and jaundice may also be present. Management is with high doses of an antithyroid drug (propylthiouracil 300–400 mg 4-hourly) given orally or via a nasogastric tube. Propranolol (80 mg 6-hourly) decreases the cardiac effects of thyroid hormones. Supportive therapy includes replacing fluid and electrolytes and cooling patients with external cooling measures. The precipitating event is identified and treated.

Myxoedema coma is a life-threatening clinical state developing in a patient with severe thyroid failure seen most commonly in an elderly patient with a longstanding history of hypothyroidism following a precipitating event such as infection, trauma, stroke, hypothermia, hypoglycaemia or drug overdose. There is deterioration in the mental status and development of absolute or relative hypothermia. Ventilatory response to hypoxia and hypercarbia is diminished, resulting in hyperventilation and CO_2 retention. The mortality rate is high. Close monitoring in the intensive care unit with cardiovascular and respiratory support is required. It is best to start with T3 5 µg intravenously or through a nasogastric tube with careful cardiac monitoring. Intravenous thyroxine is hazardous, as these patients will frequently have underlying ischaemic heart disease. Thyroxine is introduced when the dose of T3 has reached 20 µg twice-daily. Steroids may be helpful and precipitating factors should be identified and treated.

Further reading

Cooper DS. Antithyroid drugs. *N Engl J Med* 1984; **311**:1353–62.

Franklyn JA. Management of hyperthyroidism *N Engl J Med* 1994; **330**:1731–38.

Premachandra DJ, Milton CM. Cord examination after thyroidectomy. *Anaesthesia* 1989; **44**:937.

Roizen MF, Stevens A, Lampe GH. Perioperative management of patients with endocrine disease. In: Nunn JF, Utting JE, Brown BJ (eds), *General Anaesthesia*. London: Butterworths, pp. 731–8.

Sterhling L. Anaesthetic implications of hyperthyroidism. In: Brown BR (ed.), *Anaesthesia and the Patient with Endocrine Disease*. Philadelphia: FA Davis, 1980, pp. 147–58.

5 Dental anaesthesia

> What are the risks for patients associated with administration of general anaesthesia in the dental chair? How may these risks be reduced?

Anaesthesia in the dental chair poses several challenges, such as a shared airway, day-case anaesthesia and rapid turnover of cases often performed in paediatric patients.

Challenges encountered

1. Patients having come off the street directly into the dental chair must be fully starved.
2. The preoperative history must be as thorough as in hospital practice.
3. Anaesthetic monitoring is to the same standard in the dental surgery as in hospital.
4. There is a shared airway with the dental surgeon.
5. Patients are day-cases. Facility to admit patients overnight if necessary must be within reasonable reach.
6. Lack of premedication may cause greater patient anxiety, more arrhythmias under anaesthesia and a greater challenge of establishing IV access, particularly in children.
7. The airway may be obstructed by the dental pack or blood and debris. This may lead to laryngospasm.
8. Cardiac arrhythmias were much more common when halothane was in common usage. Hypoxia and hypercarbia make this complication more likely. Mostly occur during surgery and worsen during trigeminal nerve stimulation.
9. The patient's sitting position makes access to the airway more difficult.

Reducing the risk of death

The risk of death in the dental chair (1 in 250000 anaesthetics) may be reduced by:
* thorough preoperative assessment
* senior anaesthetist being present
* meticulous control of the airway using a nasal mask or, in longer cases, the LMA
* always establishing IV access.

Arrhythmias are less common with IV induction, compared with gaseous induction. Atropine increases the incidence of arrhythmias.

The *Poswillo Report* in 1990 set standards for monitoring patients undergoing sedation or general anaesthesia in the dental chair.

Further reading

Department of Health. *Poswillo Report. General Anaesthesia: Sedation and Resuscitation in Dentistry*. London: HMSO.

6 Day-case anaesthesia

> What are the advantages and disadvantages of day-case anaesthesia in patients aged more than 80 years?

Old age is associated with significant comorbidity having important implications for anaesthesia. This does not exclude elderly patients from day-case anaesthesia if their systemic disease is well controlled preoperatively.

Advantages

1. There is reduced morbidity from pneumonia, bedsores, DVT etc. with early ambulation.
2. The risk of hospital-acquired infection is reduced.
3. It may be more convenient for patients.
4. There is a cost saving for hospitals.
5. There is increased hospital efficiency.

Disadvantages

1. Coexisting disease such as hypertension, ischaemic heart disease, cerebro-vascular disease, chronic airways disease, diabetes mellitus, osteoarthritis, vision and hearing impairment are much more common in old age. Disease must be stable and well controlled.
2. Patients are at higher risk and must undergo surgery of limited complexity only.
3. It may take longer to ambulate adequately prior to going home. This may take much longer in the elderly.
4. Drug handling is slower because of the decrease in hepatic and renal function. CNS sensitivity to depressants is increased. Thus recovery from anaesthesia is slower, and the patient is less quickly 'street fit'.
5. Temperature control is impaired. This, combined with lower metabolic rate and decreased body fat, puts the elderly at risk of hypothermia and delayed recovery.
6. It may be difficult to find an accompanying responsible adult who stays with the patient overnight. The elderly often live alone with little or no family support.
7. Adequate domestic circumstances in the home must be ensured, especially access to a telephone, heating, lavatory etc.

7 Thromboembolism prophylaxis

> List the risk factors and methods for prophylaxis of venous thromboembolism in routine surgical practice.

Normally anaesthetists do not get involved in initiating prophylaxis for deep vein thrombosis. It is a serious cause of morbidity and mortality in hospital, however, with the quoted incidence of deep vein thrombosis (DVT) varying from 18% after hysterectomy to 75% after repair of fractured neck of femur. Pulmonary thromboembolism may follow DVT, this being responsible for a significant number of preventable deaths in hospital patients.

Risk factors for DVT

- *Congenital:*
  - antithrombin III deficiency
  - protein C deficiency
  - thrombophilia
  - antiphospholipid syndrome
  - protein S deficiency.
- *Acquired:*
  - family history or previous history of DVT
  - immobility
  - obesity
  - pelvic and lower-limb surgery
  - malignancy
  - varicose veins
  - oestrogen oral contraceptive pill
  - prolonged surgery.

DVT prophylaxis

Physical methods
These include:
- graduated compression stockings (TED)
- 'Flotron' boots in theatre
- early mobilisation using leg musculature as venous pumps
- pneumatic foot pumps on the ward postoperatively.

Anaesthetic technique

Regional anaesthesia is used if the block involves both legs. Thoracic epidurals for abdominal surgery do not reduce the incidence of DVTs. The mechanism of action is thought to be a combination of increased lower-limb blood flow through vasodilatation, fluid preload, less suppression of fibrinolysis compared to general anaesthesia, and reduced blood viscosity due to vasodilatation.

Pharmacological treatments

- *Unfractionated heparin* at 5000 IU subcutaneously. This is usually started before surgery (unless central neuraxial block is planned) and continued 8- to 12-hourly until discharge.
- *Low-molecular-weight heparin* (e.g. enoxaparin or tinzaparin). These have a longer duration of action and are usually prescribed once a day.

8   Patient with pacemaker

> The first patient on your operating list tomorrow morning has an implanted (perma-
> nent) cardiac pacemaker. List, with reasons, the relevant factors in your preoper-
> ative assessment.

Preoperative assessment of a patient with a permanent cardiac pacemaker
should identify what sort of pacemaker the patient has, whether it is functioning satisfactorily and whether it is being checked regularly, and what the underlying medical condition is that required it to be fitted.

Patients with pacemakers are often on cardiac medication. A detailed drug
history as well as detailed medical and anaesthetic history and assessment of
exercise tolerance are mandatory in this group of patients.

Reasons for a permanent pacemaker

- Sick sinus syndrome.
- Complete heart block.
- Tachyarrhythmias.
- Bifascicular and trifascicular block.

Pacemaker details

Type coding

Permanent pacemakers have a three- or four-letter classification:
- The chamber being paced is identified: V = ventricle, A = atrium, D = dual.
- The chamber being sensed is identified: V = ventricle, A = atrium, D = dual,
  0 = none.
- The third letter denotes the response to sensing: T = triggered. I = inhibited, D = dual, 0 = none. Thus a triggered response would pace once depolarisation was detected in the atrium or ventricle. An inhibited response
  would sense depolarisation in the atrium or ventricle and inhibit it. The
  dual mode can either trigger or inhibit sensed electrical activity; and none
  obviously implies no response when electrical activity has been detected.
- The fourth letter denotes programmability. A variable-rate pacemaker will
  be classified as R.

The latest pacemakers have a defibrillator function and have a five-letter classification.

By far the most common type of pacemaker is the VVI. This paces the ventricle, senses the ventricle, and is inhibited from pacing when R waves are
present.

Servicing details

Many patients will have a pacemaker card outlining what pacemaker they have, when it was fitted and serviced. A chest x-ray will reveal what sort of pacemaker it is via its radio-opaque code and its position.

9 Infection risk

A patient who is HIV-seropositive is scheduled to undergo laparotomy. Discuss the factors determining the risk of virus transmission to theatre staff. How can the risk be reduced?

The human immunodeficiency virus (HIV) was first identified as the causative agent for acquired immune deficiency syndrome (AIDS) in 1983. The virus is a retrovirus that targets the T-helper lymphocyte and so impairs the immune response.

The AIDS disease progresses through three stages. Seroconversion illness follows the initial HIV infection. This is a flu-like illness with sore throat, arthralgia and fever. Several years later this may be followed by persistent generalised lymphadenopathy, which then progresses to AIDS. This is characterised by opportunistic infections, Kaposi's sarcoma, lymphoma etc.

Risk of transmission of the HIV virus

HIV is mostly transmitted by blood or sexual contacts, and from mother to fetus by blood, vaginal delivery and breast milk.

- *High-risk fluids* are amniotic fluid, semen, vaginal secretions, CSF, pleural and pericardial fluid.
- *Low-risk fluids* are sputum, saliva, sweat, urine, faeces and vomit.

Compared with hepatitis B virus, HIV requires a substantial viral inoculum. The two main routes of infection are needlestick injury and entry of the virus through broken skin or mucous membranes. A hollow needlestick is likely to bear a larger inoculum compared to a solid needle. A single stab carries a 0.3% chance of infection. The risk of transmission following a splash of infected fluid on to broken skin or a mucous membrane is lower at 0.09%.

Precautions against infection

1. Use a mask, gloves and eye protection during invasive procedures. Gloves can decrease the risk of infection following needlestick injury 10–100 times.
2. Needles must not be resheathed but placed into a sharps container.
3. All open skin leasions must be covered with waterproof plasters.
4. Immediately dispose of all bodily fluids in sealed suction bottles.
5. Non-autoclavable equipment should be cleaned with 2% gluteraldehyde after the case.

Postexposure management

1. Encourage the wound to bleed and wash with soap and water.
2. Irrigate splashes on mucous membranes with copious amounts of water.
3. Active treatment with antiretroviral agents should begin 1–2 hours after exposure.

Further reading

Association of Anaesthetists. *HIV and Other Blood Borne Viruses: Guidelines for Anaesthetists*. London: AA, 1992.

10 Atrial fibrillation

An 80-year-old woman with subcapital fractured neck of femur requires surgical fixation. She is found to be in fast atrial fibrillation. What are the important points in the preoperative preparation for anaesthesia in this case?

Fast atrial fibrillation (AF) identified preoperatively may be due to a multitude of conditions. The important feature of this rhythm is whether it causes haemodynamic instability. The surgical procedure can often wait until the patient has been optimised and the rhythm either treated or at least the rate reduced. Fast AF results in increased myocardial oxygen demand and reduced myocardial oxygen supply. In non-lifesaving surgery the patient must be optimised prior to anaesthesia.

Causes of atrial fibrillation are:
- ischaemic heart disease
- thyrotoxicosis
- hypertensive cardiac disease
- chronic airways disease
- mitral valve disease
- cardiomyopathy
- congenital heart disease
- acute sepsis
- accessory conduction pathways
- alcohol excess
- idiopathic.

Treatment of AF

If the patient is haemodynamically stable, agents that slow AV conduction are used to reduce ventricular rate:
- β blockade
- calcium-channel blockers (verapamil)
- digoxin loading dose
- amiodarone.

If the patient is haemodynamically unstable, then:
- synchronised DC cardioversion starting at 100J with a light general anaesthetic.

Cardiological advice should be sought in an elderly patient such as this one for non-urgent surgery.

Multiple-choice questions: Special clinical problems

1. Recommendations to protect medical staff from AIDS include:
   a) gloves
   b) resheathing needles
   c) gowns
   d) goggles
   e) autoclaving breathing systems.

2. A man who is paraplegic because of a T4 injury is to undergo cystoscopy. A safe and effective management could be:
   a) no anaesthesia
   b) diazepam sedation
   c) local analgesia to urethra
   d) spinal (subarachnoid) block
   e) thiopentone, nitrous oxide/oxygen, halothane general anaesthetic.

3. In anaemia:
   a) P_aO_2 is reduced
   b) blood is more saturated than blood at Hb 12 g/dL
   c) 2,3-DPG is reduced
   d) blood should always be transfused prior to elective operation
   e) elective operation can satisfactorily proceed 12 hours after blood transfusion.

4. The following are associated with difficult intubations:
   a) rheumatoid arthritis
   b) ankylosing spondylitis
   c) sickle cell anaemia
   d) Marfan's syndrome
   e) acromegaly.

5. Sudden blood loss of 30% during surgery results in:
   a) immediate fall in CVP
   b) reduced urine output despite adequate maintenance of systolic BP
   c) stimulation of baroreceptors
   d) should be replaced if blood loss >15% blood volume
   e) transfusion is only required if blood pressure falls.

6. An elderly man given atropine becomes excited and confused; appropriate treatment includes:
   a) morphine
   b) physostigmine
   c) intubation and ventilation
   d) droperidol
   e) chlorpromazine.

7. In dental anaesthesia:
    a) oral debris inhalation is unlikely if the patient is supine
    b) intermittent methohexitone is a satisfactory technique for the operator anaesthetist
    c) the number of dental GAs is steadily increasing
    d) demand flow anaesthetic systems result in economy of gases
    e) simple monitoring is not essential.

8. In the elderly:
    a) systolic hypertension is common
    b) ventilatory response to CO_2 is normal
    c) P_aO_2 is less than in young adults
    d) upper-airways reflexes are impaired
    e) postoperative analgesic requirements are increased.

9. Spinal anaesthesia for fractured neck of femur repair compared with general anaesthesia:
    a) decreases mortality
    b) reduces hospital stay
    c) decreases the incidence of thromboembolism
    d) provides better immediate postoperative pain relief
    e) decreases intraoperative blood loss.

10. Goldman Cardiac Risk criteria include:
    a) previous cardiac surgery
    b) mitral valve disease
    c) hypertension
    d) atrial fibrillation
    e) previous myocardial infarction.

11. Warming blood to 37°C during massive blood transfusion:
    a) decreases the risk of citrate toxicity
    b) increases plasma potassium concentration
    c) increases plasma carbon dioxide tension
    d) decreases the incidence of arrhythmia
    e) increases CO_2 buffering capacity of cells.

12. Neuropraxia:
    a) is more common after long operations
    b) does not occur with local anaesthetics
    c) does not occur with muscle relaxants
    d) only occurs when previous neuropathy is present
    e) takes a long time to recover from.

13. Factors leading to hypothermia include:
   a) vasodilation
   b) exposure of abdominal contents
   c) neuromuscular blockers
   d) spinal anaesthesia
   e) dry gases.

14. Concerning hip arthroplasty:
   a) methyl-methacrylate is a cardiac inotrope
   b) hypoxia may be caused by marrow embolisation
   c) regional techniques are associated with a greater overall survival rate
   d) subcutaneous heparin will completely prevent DVTs
   e) hypocapnia produced by IPPV is beneficial.

15. Concerning postoperative nausea and vomiting:
   a) it is more common in women than men
   b) the incidence is 80% with general anaesthesia
   c) it is more common with thiopentone than with propofol
   d) butyrophenones can decrease the incidence
   e) it is more common with ear surgery.

16. Concerning day-case surgery:
   a) only ASA grade one patients are suitable
   b) the operation should be performed in such a way that no postoperative opiods are needed
   c) the patient should be accompanied home by an adult
   d) a laparoscopic procedure is not suitable
   e) tracheal intubation is not appropriate.

17. Agents used to decrease the pressure response to intubation include:
   a) ACE inhibitors
   b) calcium antagonists
   c) thiopentone
   d) beta-blockers
   e) fentanyl.

18. In patients with pacemakers:
   a) diathermy use should be avoided
   b) hypovolaemia is poorly tolerated
   c) electrolytes should be 'normalised' prior to surgery
   d) suxamethonium should be avoided
   e) use of volatile agents can cause deterioration of function.

19. TURP syndrome:
   a) is associated with hypokalaemia
   b) may present with convulsions
   c) is prevented by spinal anaesthesia
   d) is caused by blood loss
   e) requires treatment with diuretics.

20. The most common site of laryngeal granuloma after short-term intubation is:
    a) the piriform fossa
    b) the epiglottis
    c) anterior one-third of the vocal cords
    d) posterior one-third of the vocal cords
    e) trachea.
21. A patient with vomiting, respiratory distress, cyanosis, epigastric tenderness and subcutaneous emphysema in the neck may be suffering from:
    a) ruptured oesophagus
    b) ruptured diaphragm
    c) ruptured trachea
    d) spontaneous pneumothorax
    e) pulmonary embolus.
22. In patients with porphyria:
    a) griseofulvin may precipitate an acute attack
    b) glycine should not be used during TURP
    c) dysautonomia may occur
    d) preoperative fluid restriction is beneficial
    e) fentanyl may safely be used.
23. For a patient suffering from Parkinson's disease on L-dopa, the following agents should not be used:
    a) enflurane
    b) droperidol
    c) nitrous oxide
    d) morphine
    e) fentanyl.
24. Cricoid pressure:
    a) is effective in the presence of a nasogastric tube
    b) requires a complete cricoid cartilage to be effective
    c) should be performed with the neck extended
    d) should be performed after 5 minutes' pre-oxygenation
    e) compresses the oesphagus against the cervical vertebrae.
25. In the elderly:
    a) chest wall compliance is decreased
    b) vital capacity is decreased by 20 mL each year
    c) closing volume is less than FRC
    d) P_aO_2 is lower than in the young
    e) in a 70-year-old the alveolar/arterial oxygen difference is about 2.7 kPa.

26. The stress response to surgery may include:
    a) postoperative oliguria for 12–24 hours
    b) increased potassium excretion
    c) decreased sodium excretion
    d) increased nitrogen excretion
    e) an ebb and flow period.
27. Regarding myasthenia gravis:
    a) IgE antibodies are found in 85% of patients
    b) muscle weakness improves with exercise
    c) muscle weakness is worsened by gentamicin
    d) plasma exchange produces rapid remission
    e) thymectomy is the treatment of choice in patients over 50.
28. In the myasthenic syndrome there is:
    a) sensitivity to depolarising muscle relaxants
    b) sensitivity to non-depolarising muscle relaxants
    c) post-tetanic potentiation
    d) improvement with repeated muscle activity
    e) decreased voltages on EMG.
29. Glycine:
    a) is isotonic
    b) is used in ankylosing spondylitis
    c) is used in sickle cell anaemia
    d) is used in Marfan's syndrome
    e) is used in acromegaly.

Answers to multiple-choice questions

1.	a) True;	b) False;	c) True;	d) True;	e) False
2.	a) False;	b) False;	c) True;	d) True;	e) True
3.	a) False;	b) True;	c) False;	d) False;	e) False
4.	a) True;	b) True;	c) False;	d) True;	e) True
5.	a) True;	b) True;	c) True;	d) True;	e) False
6.	a) False;	b) True;	c) False;	d) False;	e) False
7.	a) False;	b) False;	c) False;	d) True;	e) False
8.	a) True;	b) False;	c) True;	d) True;	e) False
9.	a) False;	b) True;	c) True;	d) True;	e) True
10.	a) False;	b) False;	c) False;	d) True;	e) True
11.	a) True;	b) False;	c) False;	d) True;	e) True
12.	a) True;	b) False;	c) False;	d) False;	e) False
13.	a) True;	b) True;	c) True;	d) True;	e) True
14.	a) False;	b) True;	c) False;	d) False;	e) False
15.	a) True;	b) False;	c) True;	d) True;	e) True
16.	a) False;	b) False;	c) True;	d) False;	e) False
17.	a) True;	b) True;	c) True;	d) True;	e) True
18.	a) True;	b) True;	c) True;	d) True;	e) False
19.	a) False;	b) True;	c) False;	d) False;	e) True
20.	a) False;	b) False;	c) False;	d) True;	e) False
21.	a) True;	b) True;	c) True;	d) False;	e) False
22.	a) True;	b) False;	c) True;	d) False;	e) True
23.	a) False;	b) True;	c) False;	d) False;	e) False
24.	a) False;	b) True;	c) True;	d) False;	e) True
25.	a) True;	b) True;	c) False;	d) True;	e) True
26.	a) True;	b) True;	c) True;	d) True;	e) True
27.	a) False;	b) False;	c) True;	d) True;	e) False
28.	a) False;	b) True;	c) False;	d) True;	e) True
29.	a) True;	b) True;	c) False;	d) True;	e) True

1   Meta-analysis

> What is a meta-analysis? Outline the methodology. How are the results usually presented?

A meta-analysis is the combination of data from several studies to produce a single estimate.

Methodology

1. Before starting a meta-analysis there must be a clear definition of the question so that only studies which address this question are included.
2. All the relevant studies must be included. Which studies are included has a profound influence on the conclusions.
3. A simple literature search is not enough. Not all studies are published. Studies that produce significant differences are more likely to get published than those that do not (publication bias). Thus not only published studies must be located, but also personal knowledge of ourselves and others used to locate all the unpublished studies.
4. All available studies are scrutinised to check that they provide estimates of the same thing.
5. The original data from all the studies that fulfil the criteria for inclusion are combined into one large data file and a common estimate of the effect of the treatment or risk factor is made.
6. If the outcome measure is continuous, such as mean fall in blood pressure, analysis of variance with treatment or risk factor can be used to check that subjects are from the same population.
7. The studies cannot be combined if the treatment effect is not the same in all studies. If this is the case the studies must be examined to see whether any characteristic of the studies explains this variation. This might be a feature of the subjects, the treatment or the data collection.
8. If the data are consistent with the treatment or risk factor effect is constant, this is termed a 'fixed-effects model'.
9. If there are conflicting opposite outcomes, a single treatment effect cannot be estimated. These studies are termed a 'random-effects model'. They represent a random sample of the possible trials and estimate the mean treatment effect for that particular population. The confidence interval is usually much wider than that found using the fixed-effects model.

Meta-analysis results representation

1. If the outcome measure is dichotomous, the estimate of the treatment or risk factor effect will be in the form of an *odds ratio*.

2. Provided the odds ratios are homogeneous across studies, a common odds ratio with *confidence intervals* can be estimated. This can be done using logistic regression.
3. The data for studies where odds ratio with confidence intervals is plotted against study number is plotted on a *forest diagram*. An odds ratio for all studies represented is also plotted. For the odds ratio a logarithmic scale is often employed.

Further reading
Chalmers I, Altman DG. *Systematic Reviews*. London: BMJ Publishing, 1985.

2   Patient information sheet

> What are the main points that you would include in a patient information leaflet that you would submit to support an application to your local ethics committee to study a new non-depolarising muscle relaxant?

The patient information sheet is a requirement of ethics committees prior to a study being given approval to commence. It is a document that is given to patients prior to enrolling in a study and to take home with them after they leave hospital. Some ethics committees insist on patients being given 24 hours to reflect on the information provided in the patient information sheet prior to signing informed consent to take part in the study.

The main points that must be covered are as follows.

Study aims

What is the study investigating? This must be put in simple terms without the use of medical jargon. In this case, why study a new muscle relaxant? What are the advantages? The aim is to make it understandable to patients from all walks of life.

Who is conducting the study?

Which hospital and which department within the hospital? Researchers the patients may meet must be named. A contact telephone number must be provided in case the patient has any queries, anxieties etc.

Study design

* What is the sequence of events that the patient is likely to encounter? How many visits? What time interval? What will be done to the patient during a visit?
* How long does the study last?
* Is the muscle relaxant in question in any way harmful?
* What are the risks involved (anaphylaxis, residual block etc.)?

Patient refusal

It must be made perfectly clear that if the patient does not wish to take part in the study, or wishes to drop out of the study at any time, he or she will in no way be disadvantaged.

Financial interests

Any financial gain this study may result in must be made clear in the patient information sheet (e.g. drug company research).

It is difficult to write concise patient information sheets that are in plain English (it is said, an 8- to 10-year-old child's reading age) yet contain all the information required.

3 Evidence-based medicine

> What is evidence-based medicine? How would you apply the process to your clinical practice?

Evidence-based medicine (EBM) is the new watchword in every profession concerned with the treatment and prevention of disease.

The discipline of evidence-based medicine was introduced in the early 1990s to provide a more systematic approach to the use of evidence in making therapeutic and other decisions. Prior to this treatment strategies would often be formulated in unsystematic reviews of the published data, using selected pieces of evidence that experts in the field judged to be the most relevant or valuable. It requires both the gathering of evidence and its critical interpretation.

The emergence of EBM was made possible by:

- the development of statistical techniques for the systematic analysis of data
- the realisation that it was important to analyse all the available data, both published and unpublished
- the development of computerised databases of relevant information, linked to methods by which that information could be traced.

The tenets of EBM are that well-formulated questions about medical management can be answered by:

- carrying out high-quality, randomised, controlled clinical trials
- tracing all the available evidence
- analysing the evidence systematically
- applying the evidence to the management of the individual patient.

Application of EBM to clinical practice

The concept of 'continual learning' has recently emerged linked to continued medical education (CME). This provides a framework for clinicians to attend updates and courses that are CME-accredited. These CME-accredited modules provide a source of information where 'best practice' can be conveyed to clinicians. Furthermore, professional journals, Royal Colleges and organisations such as the Association of Anaesthetists are all vehicles to disseminate information.

Regular departmental CME meetings can provide a forum for further education and the formulation of departmental policies that encompass 'best practice' based on EBM.

The evidence on which 'best practice' is based is usually derived from large populations, which may not include patients with all the characteristics that you want answers for. There is, however, so much inter-individual variability that mean values taken from studies of populations may not be applicable to individuals. In addition there are many therapeutic problems for which adequate evidence is not available.

4   Study design for a new antiemetic drug

> You are asked to investigate the effectiveness of a new antiemetic agent. Briefly outline the principles that should guide the design of such a study.

A study investigating the effectiveness of a new antiemetic agent would investigate the drug's effectiveness over time. This would require a longitudinal study design. The other broad category of study is the cross-sectional study which describes a phenomenon fixed in time (e.g. a description of a staging system for a particular type of tumour). Every study design starts with a thorough literature review to explore previous work in the field involving the drug in question.

A prospective, randomised, controlled, double-blind trial

The gold-standard study design is said to be the prospective, randomised, controlled, double-blind trial. These terms are explained below:

* *Prospective*. This states that the study is over a defined period to examine the relative efficacy of the drug.
* *Randomised*. This is a procedure where the play of chance enters into the assignment of a subject to the alternatives under investigation. The advantage is that randomisation tends to produce study groups comparable in age, sex, bodyweight, previous history of PONV etc., as well as the actual treatment given. There are several ways of randomising patients into groups. Simple randomisation by tossing a coin or by using a random number generator is commonly used.
* *Controlled*. A control group allows the new drug to be compared with standard therapy or a placebo. A placebo is an inactive tablet or injection of a pharmacologically inert substance. Patients are ideally blinded: they are not told whether they have been given the study drug or placebo.
* *Double-blind*. The researchers are unaware what the patient has been given, either placebo or study drug. This eliminates researcher bias. Data are analysed after the study is complete when the 'code' is broken.

Study protocol

Once a study design has been decided on, a study protocol must be drawn up. The study protocol together with the patient information sheet and specimen patient consent forms are presented to the local ethics committee for approval. Ethics committees vary and there are many variations in what information the protocol must contain. Ideally the protocol outlines the following:

1. A study hypothesis – what question is this study wishing to ask?
2. Inclusion and exclusion criteria for patients – age restrictions, other medication allowable, concurrent disease etc.

3. Duration of the patient follow-up time.
4. Data collected and where it can be stored confidentially.
5. How many patients must be studied to give the study adequate power.
6. Statistical methods employed to analyse the data obtained.
7. Who will be responsible for recruiting, consenting the subjects, randomising and collecting patient data.
8. Any financial support or financial interest in the study (patients should be told this too).

Patients can be recruited into the study only after local ethics committee approval has been obtained, there has been adequate statistical preparation (preferably with expert help), a randomisation method is in place, the drug and placebo are available, and it has been decided what data to collect.

5   Data interpretation

> The plasma concentrations of a drug have been measured in 20 normal patients and in 20 patients with renal failure. What simple statistical tests exist to determine whether these two sets of observations differ at the 5% level of significance? What assumptions are inherent in each test you describe?

Data

1. The trial in question is a longitudinal prospective study.
2. The data to be interpreted are plasma concentration of a drug. This is thus termed quantitative or numerical data rather than qualitative or nominal data. Nominal data are data one can name (e.g. male or female, dead or alive). Within the broad classification of numerical data, the data can be subclassified as numerical continuous data: the data can take any value within a given range.

Statistical tests

1. The data are a small sample of continuous data. Patients have concentrations of drug measured at a specific time interval and the difference compared to baseline. Thus we are dealing with paired data and the paired t-test can be applied.
2. Student's t-test is another statistical test that can be used for small samples of continuous data.

Assumptions made

The paired t-test and Student's t-test are both parametric tests that make the assumption that the *data are taken from a normal population with a normal distribution*. In the case of the paired t-test, the assumption is that the difference in values measured compared to baseline follows a normal distribution rather than the basic observations. A normal distribution is the histogram of a continuous variable obtained from a single measurement on different subjects which has a characteristic 'bell-shape'.

The calculation of a significance level of 5% means that there is a 5% chance of the difference measured being due to chance. This hypothesis testing is a method of deciding whether the data are consistent with the *null hypothesis*. The null hypothesis assumes that there is no difference between groups; i.e. no difference in blood drug level in patients with renal failure compared to patients with normal renal function.

Further reading
Campbell MJ, Machin D. *Medical Statistics: a Commonsense Approach*, 3rd edn. Chichester: John Wiley.

Multiple-choice questions: Study design and statistics

1. Concerning exponential decay:
   a) half time constant equals a half litre
   b) $3 \times$ time constant equals 97%
   c) the rate of change is proportional to the quantity at a certain time
   d) at one time constant, 37% remains
   e) the time constant is the time at which the process would have been complete had the initial rate of change continued.

2. In statistics, $p < 0.001$:
   a) means that there is a less than 1 in 1000 chance that the difference could be due to chance
   b) rejects the null hypothesis
   c) means that the data are normally distributed
   d) the difference is statistically significant
   e) the difference is clinically significant.

3. In a controlled trial to compare two treatments, randomisation is undertaken because:
   a) the clinician does not know which treatment group patients are allocated to
   b) the two groups will be similar in disease severity
   c) the clinician knows which treatment patients receive
   d) the number of patients in each group is identical
   e) the sample may be referred to a known population.

4. As the size of a random sample increases:
   a) the standard deviation decreases
   b) the standard error of the mean decreases
   c) the mean decreases
   d) the range is likely to increase
   e) the accuracy of the parameter estimates increases.

5. A 95% confidence interval for a mean:
   a) is wider than a 99% confidence interval
   b) in repeated samples will include the population mean 95% of the time
   c) will include the sample mean with a probability of 1
   d) is a useful way of describing the accuracy of a study
   e) will include 95% of the observations of a sample.

6. The *p* value:
    a) is the probability that the null hypothesis is false
    b) is large for small studies
    c) is the probability of the observed result, or one more extreme, if the null hypothesis were true
    d) can be any value less than 1
    e) can be more than 1.
7. A correlation coefficient:
    a) always lies in the range 0 to 100
    b) could be used to examine the relationship between urea concentration and creatinine clearance in a sample of the population
    c) is a means of measuring the relationship between two variables
    d) can be used to predict one variable from another
    e) can have a negative value.
8. In a normal distribution:
    a) the mean, the median and the modal values are coincident
    b) there is no skew of the curve
    c) 75% of all values lie within one standard deviation of the mean
    d) about two-thirds of all values occur within one standard deviation greater or less than the mean value
    e) there are more values positive to the modal value than negative.
9. The standard deviation of a group of data:
    a) is the square of the variance
    b) is a measure of central tendency
    c) is in the same units as the original data
    d) for normally distributed values is used to predict relative frequencies
    e) is independent of the mean value of the data.
10. In an exponentially changing process:
    a) the time constant is twice the half-time
    b) the time constant is half the time taken
    c) the time constant is 37% of the change
    d) by 3 time constants 95% of the change will have occurred
    e) the rate of change is by constant proportions.
11. In clinical trials patients can be assigned to comparable groups by:
    a) tossing a coin
    b) order of presentation
    c) *p* value
    d) chi-squared test
    e) random number tables.

Answers to multiple-choice questions

1. a) False;   b) True;   c) True;   d) True;   e) True
2. a) True;   b) True;   c) False;   d) True;   e) False
3. a) False;   b) True;   c) False;   d) False;   e) False
4. a) False;   b) True;   c) False;   d) True;   e) True
5. a) False;   b) True;   c) True;   d) True;   e) False
6. a) False;   b) False;   c) True;   d) True;   e) False
7. a) False;   b) False;   c) True;   d) False;   e) True
8. a) True;   b) True;   c) False;   d) True;   e) False
9. a) False;   b) False;   c) True;   d) True;   e) False
10. a) False;   b) False;   c) False;   d) True;   e) True
11. a) True;   b) True;   c) False;   d) False;   e) True

1 Propofol versus thiopentone

Compare the pharmacology of propofol and thiopentone.

Propofol and thiopentone are the two most commonly used intravenous induction agents. Propofol has in recent years eclipsed thiopentone because of its better side-effect profile and ease of use, and its use in total intravenous anaesthesia.

Presentation

Thiopentone (thiopental sodium) is the sulphur analogue of pentobarbital and is presented as a yellowish powder with a bitter taste and faint smell of garlic. It is stored in nitrogen to prevent chemical reaction with atmospheric carbon dioxide, and mixed with 6% anhydrous sodium carbonate to increase its solubility in water. It is available as single-dose ampoules of 500 mg and is dissolved in distilled water to produce a 2.5% solution which will remain usable for 24 hours.

Propofol is formulated in a white, aqueous emulsion containing soyabean oil and purified egg phosphatide. Ampoules of the drug contain 200 mg of propofol in 20 mL (1% solution) and 50 mL bottles containing 1% or 2% solutions.

Pharmacodynamics

Central nervous system

Thiopentone produces anaesthesia in one arm–brain circulation. The cerebral metabolic rate is reduced, with secondary decreases in cerebral blood volume and intracranial pressure. There is acute tolerance to thiopentone with recovery of consciousness occurring at higher blood concentrations if a large dose is given. The drug has an antanalgesic effect and reduces the pain threshold. Thiopentone is a very potent anticonvulsant.

Propofol, too, induces anaesthesia in one arm–brain circulation. Transfer of the drug to the sites of action in the brain is slightly slower compared to thiopentone. There is a delay in the loss of eyelash reflex. Cerebral metabolic rate, cerebral blood flow and intracranial pressure are reduced. Although EEG frequency decreases and amplitude increases, there is no evidence that propofol induces seizures.

Cardiovascular system

Thiopentone depresses myocardial contractility and causes peripheral vasodilatation. Blood pressure drops, but profound hypotension may occur in the presence of hypovolaemia or cardiac disease.

Arterial pressure decreases to a greater extent with propofol. There is a slight reduction in myocardial contractility, but the main reduction in blood pressure is due to peripheral vasodilatation. The degree of hypotension is related to the speed of administration of propofol. Propofol should thus be administered slowly in the elderly and frail.

Respiratory system
With thiopentone, a short period of apnoea is followed by a few deep breaths. Ventilatory drive is reduced owing to decreased sensitivity of the respiratory centre to carbon dioxide. There is an increase in bronchial muscle tone, but bronchospasm is very uncommon. Upper-airway reflexes are heightened and laryngeal spasm can be precipitated by the presence of secretions, blood or an airway device in the airway as well as by surgical stimulation.

With propofol, apnoea occurs for a longer period after induction of anaesthesia. Propofol also causes a decreased ventilatory response to carbon dioxide. Propofol has no effect on bronchial smooth muscle. Unlike thiopentone, propofol suppresses laryngeal reflexes.

Other systems
Skeletal muscle tone is reduced with both drugs. Thiopentone crosses the placenta readily but fetal levels do not reach maternal drug levels. Propofol is usually not used for rapid-sequence induction in obstetric anaesthesia as its safety to the neonate has not been established. Intraocular pressure is reduced and eye reflexes (corneal, conjunctival, eyelash and eyelid) are abolished.

Pharmacokinetics

About 80% of thiopentone is bound to albumin in the blood. More free drug is available in hypoalbuminaemic conditions (liver failure, malnutrition). Thiopentone is very lipid-soluble and predominately un-ionized at body pH. Thiopentone metabolism occurs predominately in the liver with metabolites being excreted in the kidneys. The terminal elimination half-life is approximately 11.5 hours; 10–15% of the remaining drug is metabolised each hour. A hangover effect is common as up to 30% of the drug may remain in the body after 24 hours. Elimination is impaired in the elderly, and dosage should be based on lean body mass in obese patients.

Similar to thiopentone, propofol is distributed rapidly and blood concentrations decline exponentially. Metabolism is mainly in the liver although extra-hepatic sites are involved in metabolism to a minor degree. The kidneys excrete the metabolites as glucuronides. The terminal elimination half-life of propofol is 3–5 hours, which is considerably faster than thiopentone.

2 Therapeutic uses of magnesium

> What are the therapeutic uses of magnesium and how does it work?

Magnesium is a drug that has been put to increasing therapeutic use recently. It is an important intracellular cation and is an important constituent of human body enzyme systems.

Therapeutic uses

- *Acute arrhythmias.* It is the treatment of choice for torsade de pointes (a type of ventricular tachycardia occasionally induced by class 1a or class 3 antiarrhythmic drugs). It is used to treat tachyarrhythmias, particularly those induced by digitalis, bupivacaine or adrenaline (i.e. iatrogenic). Magnesium causes widening of the QRS with a prolonged P-Q interval.
- *Pre-eclampsia and eclampsia.* Magnesium sulphate decreases systemic vascular resistance and so reduces blood pressure. It also reduces CNS excitability and can be used to pre-empt eclamptic convulsions.
- *In the ICU.* Magnesium is used in critical illness to treat nutritional deficiency and malabsorption syndromes. It can be infused in patients with tetanus to treat muscle spasm and autonomic instability.
- *Acute severe asthma.*

Actions of magnesium sulphate

Magnesium has an important role in the regulation of cellular functions, and magnesium ions antagonise calcium ions. The action of magnesium – which accounts for most of its effects – is to inhibit calcium ion influx into cells through calcium channels owing to high intracellular magnesium ion levels. Magnesium also inhibits the release of catecholamines and so has an antiadrenergic action.

Further reading

Which anticonvulsant for eclampsia? Evidence from the Collaborative Eclampsia Trial. *Lancet* 1995; **345**:1455–63.

3   Use of nitrous oxide (N$_2$O)

> Discuss the reasons for and against the use of nitrous oxide in anaesthetic prac-
> tice.

Nitrous oxide is the oldest anaesthetic agent used in modern anaesthetic practice. Its place in current anaesthetic practice is under scrutiny with the availability of new fast-onset and fast-offset opiates with far fewer side-effects.

Advantages of nitrous oxide

1. It is a potent analgesic. The analgesic effect is due to direct action on opiate
   receptors, and indirectly by release of endogenous opiates.
2. It is a carrier gas for volatile anaesthetic agents.
3. There is rapid onset and rapid offset due to the low blood/gas partition
   coefficient of 0.47.
4. Onset of anaesthesia is accelerated due to the second-gas effect. This is particularly noticeable during gas induction of anaesthesia in children.

Disadvantages of nitrous oxide

1. Diffusion hypoxia is a problem owing to rapid washout of nitrous oxide
   into the alveoli resulting in a low partial pressure of oxygen. Supplemental
   oxygen is required for 10–15 minutes.
2. It has an emetic effect leading to nausea and vomiting. It has a direct effect
   on opioid receptors. The emetic effect is also possibly due to gastric distension.
3. It is a cardiovascular depressant. There is a direct negative inotropic and
   chronotropic effect. This is particularly marked if cardiac function is
   already compromised, as in ischaemic heart disease or sepsis.
4. It has an increased diffusion capacity compared to nitrogen. This leads to
   air-filled spaces becoming expanded (middle ear, nasal sinuses, bowel,
   vitreo-retinal work, pneumothorax, ETT cuffs, air embolus, bullae).
5. Bone marrow toxicity is a potential problem. Nitrous oxide oxidises the
   cobalt atom in vitamin B$_{12}$. Vitamin B$_{12}$ is a co-factor for the enzyme
   methionine synthetase. Lack of methionine synthetase leads to impaired
   formation of tetrahydrofolate which is an important substrate involved in
   nucleotide and DNA synthesis. This thus leads to megaloblastic anaemia
   following prolonged exposure to NO. The same mechanism may lead to
   teratogenicity.
6. Being a 'greenhouse gas', nitrous oxide is an environment pollutant.

4   Anaesthetic implications of substance-abusing patients

> Outline the problems involved in anaesthetising an intravenous heroin abuser needing urgent surgery for incision of perianal abscess.

Drug-dependent patients presenting for both emergency and routine surgery are becoming increasingly common. These patients can provide considerable challenges to the anaesthetist.

Substances abused

It is often extremely difficult to obtain accurate information from these patients. It is important to try to build up a rapport. This group of patients can be extremely manipulative, however.

Drugs abused vary widely. Amphetamines (ecstasy), cannabis, cocaine, benzodiazepines, opiates and solvents (glue) are the most common.

General medical condition

Coexisting disease such as myocarditis, endocarditis and bacteraemia should be sought. These may occur due to the introduction of pathogens via contaminated needles and infected venepuncture sites.

Patients often have a poor nutritional state and poor oral hygiene. Concomitant alcohol abuse can lead to global cardiomyopathy, pulmonary hypertension and arrhythmias. There may be anaemia due to poor nutrition and/or gastrointestinal blood loss.

Hepatic insufficiency may be due to coexisting infection with hepatitis B or C. Alcoholic liver disease may lead to protein deficiency, in particular albumin, plasma cholinesterase and clotting factors.

Specific problems

Sudden drug withdrawal whilst in hospital leads to acute autonomic hyperactivity. Specialist advice must be sought. Withdrawing opiates from these patients is not the correct way to proceed. Patients should receive their regular script as they normally would out of hospital (e.g. methadone).

Severe alcohol withdrawal occurs 12–36 hours following abstention and can manifest itself as delirium tremens, autonomic hyperactivity, abdominal pain, diarrhoea and agitation. Acute alcohol withdrawal can be treated with benzodiazepines.

Anaesthetic management

1. Venous access may be impossible peripherally. In this case, central venous access should be sought.
2. Regional anaesthesia should be used where at all possible for postoperative pain relief, to avoid opiate use.
3. Intraoperative doses of opiates required are likely to be much higher than in non-dependent patients.
4. Ward staff must be asked to involve the acute pain team early on to bring consistency to the postoperative pain management plan.
5. Acute withdrawal may occur in the postoperative period.

5 Drugs used to induce hypotension

> Classify, giving examples and mode of action, the drugs used in anaesthetic prac-
> tice to induce hypotension deliberately.

Volatile anaesthetic agents

Isoflurane causes hypotension as a result of peripheral vasodilation without
effecting myocardial contractility. In higher doses, CNS depression prevents
reflex tachycardia.

The older volatile agents such as halothane and enflurane cause myocardial
depression as well as peripheral vasodilation.

Alpha-adrenoceptor blockers

Phentolamine and phenoxybenzamine produce competitive blockade of sympathetic postsynaptic noradrenergic receptors. Phenoxybenzamine is usually
used preoperatively for several weeks to control chronic hypertension in
patients with conditions such as phaeochromocytoma. Phentolamine has a
rapid onset lasting 15–20 minutes. It reduces blood pressue via α_1 block, so
decreasing peripheral resistance. There is also weak β sympathomimetic activity.

Beta-adrenoceptor blockers

Beta-blockers reduce cardiac output and heart rate. There may be some action
on the renin–angiotensin system. All are competitive antagonists but have
varying receptor selectivity. Esmolol is a short-acting drug that can be given IV
intraoperatively.

Alpha$_2$-adrenoceptor agonists

Clonidine acts centrally by reducing sympathetic outflow. Clonidine has analgesic and sedative properties.

Direct vasodilators

Sodium nitroprusside (SNP) dilates resistance and capacitance vessels. Its mode
of action is via nitric oxide. SNP increases cerebral blood flow and intracranial
pressure. There is rapid onset and offset (2–3 minutes). Metabolism creates
cyanide ions which irreversibly bind to cytochrome oxidase at levels above
8 μg/kg/min.

Glyceryl trinitrate (GTN) causes slower reduction and recovery in blood
pressue. GTN dilates capacitance vessels with little or no effect on resistance
vessels. It has a greater effect on systolic compared to diastolic pressure. GTN

increases cerebral blood flow and intracranial pressure. It mediates hypotensive action via nitric oxide and cyclic GMP within cells, decreasing available calcium ions.

Hydralazine's action is also mediated via an increase in cyclic GMP and reduced calcium ion availability. Hydralazine mainly reduces arteriolar tone with some effect on venous tone. Reflex tachycardia sometimes occurs with this agent.

Ganglion blockers
Trimetaphan blocks nicotinic receptors at autonomic ganglia (both sympathetic and parasympathetic). There is no effect on nicotinic receptors at the neuromuscular junction. There is a reduction in cardiac contractility. A reflex tachycardia is common and causes histamine release. There is marked tachyphylaxis, and hypoxic pulmonary vasoconstriction is reversed.

6   Postoperative nausea and vomiting (PONV)

Describe the principles underlying the treatment of postoperative nausea and vomiting (PONV).

Forty per cent of all surgical patients experience PONV. There are certain patient factors as well as certain operations that make PONV more likely.

Factors

Patient factors

1. Past history of PONV.
2. History of motion sickness.
3. Obesity.
4. Female.
5. Early ambulation.
6. Children.

Surgical factors

1. Gastrointestinal surgery.
2. Gynaecological surgery.
3. ENT (blood in stomach), middle ear.
4. Extraocular muscle surgery.
5. Emergency surgery (full stomach).

Pharmacological factors

1. Opiate analgesics.
2. Volatile anaesthetic agents.
3. Etomidate, thiopentone.
4. Hypotension.
5. Nitrous oxide.

Miscellaneous factors

1. Prolonged fasting.
2. Pain.
3. Fear.
4. Excessive pharyngeal manipulation.
5. Hypoglycaemia.
6. Uraemia.

Treatment of PONV

The focus is initially on avoiding or preventing metabolic causes (dehydration, hypoglycaemia), fear, pain and prolonged fasting.

Anaesthetic technique can go a long way to avoiding PONV. In high-risk patients, opiates, volatile agents, nitrous oxide, thiopentone and etomidate can be avoided in favour of a propofol-based totally intravenous anaesthetic (TIVA). Propofol has intrinsic antiemetic properties.

Pharmacological treatment is aimed at targeting a number of different receptor types which are linked to the vomiting centre in the reticular formation of the medulla within the blood–brain barrier. The vomiting centre receives afferents from the chemoreceptor trigger zone situated in the area postrema in the floor of the fourth ventricle:

* *Serotonin* (5-hydroxytryptamine) *receptors*. Ondansetron and granesetron antagonise 5HT receptors found predominately in the gut.
* *Dopamine* (D2) *receptors*. Droperidol and metaclopramide act on dopamine receptors found in the chemoreceptor trigger zone and influence vagal afferents.
* *Histamine* (H1) *receptors*. These are antagonised by cyclizine and to a lesser extent droperidol. They are situated mainly in the vestibular labyrinth.
* *Cholinergic* (muscurinic) *receptors*. Hyoscine, glycopyrrolate and atropine antagonise these receptors found in the vestibular labyrinth and chemoreceptor trigger zone.
* *Non-specific action*. There are a number of drugs like propofol that have an antiemetic action but where the site of action is unclear. Dexamethasone similarly has an antiemetic action and is often used in paediatric anaesthesia. Recent interest in cannabinoids may yield a new group of antiemetics.

Further reading

Anaesthesia 1994; **49** (supplement).

Strunin L, Rowbotham D, Miles A (eds). *The Effective Management of Postoperative Nausea and Vomiting*. Aesculapius Press, 1999.

Multiple-choice questions: Applied pharmacology

1. Propofol:
   a) is suspended in an emulsion of soyabean oil and egg phosphatide
   b) can produce green urine
   c) has little effect on the cardiovascular system
   d) impairs ventilatory response to CO_2
   e) has no effect on intraocular pressure.
2. The following are safe in porphyria:
   a) morphine
   b) sulphonamides
   c) chlorpromazine
   d) barbiturates
   e) diazepam.
3. If 50% nitrous oxide is inhaled for 3 days:
   a) the lymphocyte count falls
   b) methionine synthetase activity is reduced
   c) megaloblastic bone marrow changes occur
   d) B_{12} deficiency anaemia develops
   e) peripheral neuropathy develops.
4. Halothane hepatotoxicity is linked to:
   a) age
   b) obesity
   c) prolonged anaesthesia
   d) a history of cholecystitis
   e) hypoxia.
5. Isoflurane:
   a) has a similar boiling point to enflurane
   b) has a similar saturated vapour pressure to halothane
   c) has a lower blood/gas coefficient than halothane
   d) is extensively metabolised
   e) has a MAC of 0.56% in oxygen.
6. Cerebral vascular resistance is reduced by:
   a) halothane
   b) enflurane
   c) isoflurane
   d) trichloroethylene (trilene)
   e) thiopentone.

7. Methohexitone:
   a) has a pH less than 8 in 1% solution
   b) is a methylated thiobarbiturate
   c) has a longer duration of action than thiopentone
   d) does not cause pain on injection
   e) is associated with fewer excitatory phenomena than thiopentone.
8. Increase in K^+ needing treatment may occur:
   a) after cardiac bypass
   b) in diabetic coma
   c) after suxamethonium administration
   d) after severe burns
   e) after severe tissue damage.
9. The pressor response to intubation may be attenuated by:
   a) calcium-channel blockers
   b) thiopentone
   c) fentanyl
   d) angiotension-converting enzyme inhibitors
   e) beta-blockers.
10. The oculocardiac reflex is prevented by:
    a) atropine
    b) small increments of isoprenaline
    c) retrobulbar block
    d) deep anaesthesia
    e) avoidance of traction on extraocular muscles.
11. The MAC of isoflurane:
    a) decreases with age
    b) is decreased with acute alcohol intake
    c) is lower in men than women
    d) is higher in neonates compared to a 2-year-old
    e) is decreased in pregnancy.
12. The sympathoadrenal axis may be stimulated by:
    a) etomidate
    b) cyclopropane
    c) halothane
    d) methoxyflurane
    e) di-ethyl ether.
13. Following intravenous thiopentone and suxamethonium, causes of lack of muscle relaxation include:
    a) drug interaction
    b) subcutaneous inactivation
    c) porphyria
    d) malignant hyperpyrexia
    e) myotonia congenita.

14. Concerning analgesic drugs:
    a) paracetamol is an anti-inflammatory drug
    b) toxic doses of aspirin increase the rate and depth of respirations
    c) aspirin-like drugs shorten time for delivery of a fetus
    d) indomethacin lowers a raised body temperature
    e) aspirin displaces other drugs from plasma proteins.

15. Concerning analgesic drugs:
    a) indomethacin is an addictive drug
    b) paracetamol causes gastric irritation
    c) unionised acetylsalicylic acid is absorbed more readily than the ionised form
    d) the analgesic properties of indomethacin are best seen when pain is associated with inflammation
    e) phenylbutazone is the drug of choice for headache.

16. The following drugs may be safely used in porphyria:
    a) barbiturates
    b) bupivacaine
    c) lignocaine
    d) chlorpromazine
    e) sulphonamides.

Answers to multiple-choice questions

1.	a) True;	b) True;	c) False;	d) True;	e) False
2.	a) True;	b) False;	c) True;	d) False;	e) True
3.	a) False;	b) True;	c) True;	d) False;	e) False
4.	a) False;	b) True;	c) False;	d) False;	e) True
5.	a) False;	b) True;	c) True;	d) False;	e) False
6.	a) True;	b) True;	c) True;	d) True;	e) False
7.	a) False;	b) False;	c) False;	d) False;	e) False
8.	a) True;	b) True;	c) False;	d) True;	e) True
9.	a) True;	b) True;	c) True;	d) False;	e) True
10.	a) True;	b) False;	c) True;	d) True;	e) True
11.	a) True;	b) True;	c) False;	d) False;	e) True
12.	a) False;	b) True;	c) False;	d) False;	e) True
13.	a) True;	b) True;	c) False;	d) True;	e) True
14.	a) False;	b) True;	c) False;	d) True;	e) True
15.	a) False;	b) False;	c) False;	d) True;	e) False
16.	a) False;	b) True;	c) True;	d) True;	e) False

Index

Page numbers in **bold** type relate to the main subjects of short-answer questions; those in *italics* refer to multiple-choice questions. Answers to the multiple-choice questions are not included in the index, but they may be found immediately after the questions at the end of each section.